The
ANIMALS NEVER LIE

BARB FOX, DVM

The Animals Never Lie

Barbara Fox, DVM

She may be reached at *drbfox@yahoo.com*

And please visit *www.barbfoxdvm.com*

Cover photo from 123RF.com

Back Cover and interior photos from Barb Fox

Cover and book layout by Laura Ashton
laura@gitflorida.com

ISBN: 978-1983950483

Printed in the United States of America

Disclaimer

This book is not intended to be used to diagnose, treat, cure, or heal. It is simply a compilation of case reports from Dr. Fox's holistic veterinary office where a combination of natural and conventional therapies have been used in various animal species. The book is to be used for educational purposes only.

If your animal has an injury, illness, or disease of any kind, please consult with your veterinarian and obtain appropriate diagnostic testing and treatment.

The author accepts no responsibility for those who have attempted self-diagnosis or who have tried to duplicate a scenario from this book to attempt treatment on their own animals.

The use of alternative therapies has real value in supporting, promoting, and maintaining the body's organ systems. Because most of the therapies described in this book are not FDA-approved, Dr. Fox makes no claims as to their efficacy or ability to eradicate, alleviate, or treat specific diseases.

Other Books by Dr. Fox

The Infinite Bond - 2017

Dedication

*To the many animals who have made me
wiser, more humble, have filled me with
love, have made me laugh, and who have
taught me more than I ever could have
imagined, I dedicate this book to you.*

Preface

So many people ask me why and how I got into holistic veterinary medicine. After all, I had been in conventional practice for thirteen years. Why change now? The answer is two-fold: I was frustrated seeing patients coming back for the same issues over and over without any kind of long-lasting resolution of their symptoms. More importantly, though, was my own health scare. I was diagnosed with an aggressive breast cancer in 2007.

The day I heard the word "cancer" was one of the worst of my entire life. You're always in denial, thinking it will happen to someone else. That "someone else" was now *me*. I sat in the doctor's office with pounding heart and shaking fingers while the gynecologist quietly pointed out the mass on the mammogram, its ugly tentacles probing deep into my right breast tissue. All I could think was, *This looks like a Tazmanian devil on steroids.* My immediate thought was to slice this demonic clump of cells out of my body as fast as possible.

As I listened to the physician explain treatment options, my mind went numb. My mother had passed away from terrible side effects of treatment when she was diagnosed with a rare form of uterine cancer just four years prior. The doctor's grim and sorrowful expression told me everything I didn't want to acknowledge as I felt my pulse bounding and a queasy feeling overtaking my stomach. *Do they all have that pitiful look?* I wondered. *There isn't a flicker of hope written anywhere on her face.* She'd seen too much of this disease: the dreams that were lost, the fear on her patients' faces, the families turned upside down, the weariness from fighting a wicked disease.

The gynecologist referred me to a general surgeon to confirm the diagnosis with a needle biopsy, even though it was blatantly obvious to me that the mass was malignant. I'd seen too many radiographs of dogs and cats with aggressive carcinomas that looked exactly like my mammogram. That same day, I nervously followed the thin, yellow strip taped to the hospital floor to the radiology department, where I met with the surgeon who would take a small sample of breast tissue using an ultrasound to locate the rogue mass. The pathology report confirmed the diagnosis: ductal adenocarcinoma.

At the time, I was plagued with other health issues. I had just turned fifty years of age, and for the past thirty years had suffered from fibromyalgia, asthma, severe allergies, and nagging acid reflux. I just knew intuitively that radiation and chemotherapy would end my life prematurely. In fact, I was more frightened of conventional treatment than the cancer. Knowing I had been in anaphylactic shock, a life-threatening allergic reaction, on three different occasions, I was convinced the chemo drugs would kill me. Furthermore, the thought of subjecting my body to radiation just didn't seem like a logical plan. Healthy x-ray technicians and radiographers protected themselves from the harmful rays with neck to knee lead aprons, thyroid collars, and specialized eyewear. And here I was—an already unhealthy person— being blasted with radiation.

I drove home that afternoon with a script running through my head of what I was going to tell my husband. Gary's mother had died of breast cancer years prior to our meeting, and I knew he wouldn't take this news well. We had only been married for three years after both of us had endured painful divorces. Now that we were so incredibly happy together, how would I tell the love of my life that I had a living, growing aggregation of malicious cells in my breast that wasn't there a month ago when I had my annual checkup? How would I convince him to support me with whatever decision I made about my treatment?

Through a lot of prayer, soul-searching, and research, I chose *not* to go through conventional therapy. Instead, I elected to have only the mass removed, keeping my breast and all of the associated lymph nodes. I read many books written by cancer survivors, and the main theme was that all of them had a "pitbull" type of determination to live, regardless of what treatments they chose (or declined). It was fascinating to learn that people with cancers of all types could survive, given the right mindset and "tools" from nature to bring the body back into balance, even those with a stage four diagnosis.

Gary was understandably frightened with my decision. Actually, he was scared out of his wits that I wanted to try to heal my body without chemo and radiation. After I explained my fears about how the drugs and radiation would affect my body, he reluctantly agreed with me and eventually gave me his blessing. As he read books and watched videos featuring people who'd survived cancer after choosing a holistic approach to their treatments, he became more comfortable with the decision.

When I was in the recovery room after having the lumpectomy, the surgeon met with Gary. He said the mass had a strange "capsule" around it, like the body was trying to wall the cancer off. (Little did he know that a week before surgery, I had a very gifted healer perform an energy session on me, asking the body to gather up the cancer cells so the surgeon could remove it in its entirety.) The surgeon hesitantly gave me the option of foregoing chemotherapy, since the tumor was pretty well contained and it was just at the cutoff of 2.0 centimes in diameter. But he was adamant that I'd need radiation. He really pushed for six weeks of therapy, five days a week, at a clinic located a little over two hours from home. I had already done my own research on radiation therapy, and I was surprised beyond belief to find out that the mortality rate for women with breast cancer was exactly the same after fifteen years, whether they went through radiation or not. When I showed the research paper to the surgeon, he looked at me and said, "I can't argue with that." I then signed a paper confirming that I declined the treatment he recommended.

What I *did* plan was to change my mindset. I adopted an attitude of gratitude for everything, even the cancer. Yes, you read that correctly. Had I not had the cancer "scare," I would not have turned on to holistic medicine. Nor would I have grown emotionally and spiritually as I have in the past decade. I wouldn't be here helping my animal patients nor would I be teaching others that there *is* another way to treat the body.

I also cleaned up my diet, eating organically as possible and incorporating high quality nutritional supplements into my regimen. After reading countless articles on the myriad benefits of whole food supplements, enzymes, and phytonutrients, I was convinced lots of diseases could be alleviated with diet and exercise alone. Although I already worked out several days a week, I ramped up the intensity to increase circulation and sweat out the toxins secretly residing in my body.

Stress can play a huge part in suppression or overstimulation of the immune system, altering its vibrational frequency (a term used in quantum physics), consequently opening up the body for immune-mediated or auto-immune assaults. Twenty years of enduring a difficult and emotionally draining marriage took a good toll on my health. Although the tumor wasn't detected until it had reached two centimeters in diameter, its growth started many years before I ended our dysfunctional relationship. With the help of essential oils that were emotionally balancing, support from good friends and healing practitioners, and assistance from our Creator, I was able to release the past hurts and insults.

I was initially introduced to essential oils from a large animal colleague who practiced in a neighboring community. I'd heard of essential oils, although I thought they were just for "smelling good" and didn't realize that pure, genuine oils had medicinal qualities until I started attending classes locally. Dr. Merlin, the host for the class, showed me research papers that discussed how certain essential oils, such as frankincense, contained compounds such as boswellic acids that caused cancer cell *apoptosis* (death of unhealthy cells) as well as suppressing tumor growth and improving the overall immune response. That information had me hooked. I wanted to learn how essential oils could help my body become healthy again. Dr. Merlin directed me to legitimate research sites where I could study the science behind the oils.

Fortunately, a friend of mine told me about a chiropractor that performed a technique called Contact Reflex Analysis. CRA helps find imbalances in the body so proper nutritional supplements and other modalities could be utilized in balancing the various organ systems. When I filled out the initial paperwork and handed it to the CRA chiropractor, she looked at my medical history with a neutral expression on her face. She then leaned toward me and put her hand over mine in a comforting manner, and said with a genuine smile, "I see we have a temporary health challenge. Let's get started."

Her voice was so confident, yet so gentle. *A temporary health challenge?! Wow, the gynecologist's office already had me dead and buried!* The sight of the doctor's face when she gave me the news flashed across my mind. Comparing her expression to the one in front of me now made me certain I'd come to the right place.

Over the course of a year and a half, the old maladies like muscle pain, digestive issues, allergies, and respiratory issues fell by the wayside. I felt better than I had in the past twenty years. Was the cancer gone? I believed wholeheartedly that yes, it was gone. Once you set your mind to have an undeniable, rock-solid belief system, your body will respond. Did I go back for yearly or semi-annual mammograms? No. But why not, you might ask?

First of all, if there was a suspicious area indicated on the mammogram, I would have been sent directly to the radiology department for an ultrasound-guided biopsy. That's where the doctor injects a local anesthetic directly into the breast tissue to numb it. Then a long, thick needle is inserted through the skin and into the suspicious area. Hopefully, after a few probing movements, there will be enough sample in the end of the biopsy needle to extract and send to the pathology department for analysis. Although the probability is remote, there is a chance that damage from the biopsy needle may trigger faster growth in an existing cyst or tumor (though you won't hear mainstream medicine mentioning this possibility). Secondly, mammograms press firmly on delicate breast tissue, possibly causing trauma, especially where scar tissue may have formed. Thirdly, mammograms are ionizing radiation (x-rays), and subjecting myself to radiation on a regular basis didn't jive with me.

I chose a totally different path to make sure the "c" never reared its ugly head again, so I didn't have to feel pressured to have a mammogram every stinking year. So I could go forth with life fearlessly. So I could pay it forward for being blessed with abundant health and wellness.

Faith is a huge thing with me. I talked with God *a lot* when I was setting my mind to envision my body completely whole and healthy again.

But my conversations always focused on gratitude and thanksgiving for the amazing healing that had come my way, never *hoping* to be healed or *asking* for a "cancer-free" body, because that would imply that I didn't believe it *could* happen. I had to say, without a sliver of doubt, that, *"I am healed. Thank you dear God for Your love and healing energy."*

Because of the miracles I had now experienced using *natural* modalities and God's beautiful grace, I started looking into how I could improve my animal patients' lives with the same kinds of things (nutrition, essential oils, herbs, homeopathics, energy work). I joined the American Holistic Veterinary Medical Association and attended as many alternative and holistic conferences as I could. (I still attend as many as I can afford). Our own animals became "practice" models, trying things on them to see what response I got before recommending them to my clients. The results have been absolutely phenomenal.

I now had another "toolbox" to share with my precious animal patients and their guardians.

– Barb Fox, DVM

Introduction

"Why does my dog still itch so badly after he goes off of prednisone and antibiotics?"

"Doctor, I'm so afraid to have my dog go through surgery at her age."

"I can't bear the thought of putting my horse down because of an injured tendon. Please help me."

"I don't want to put my cat through chemotherapy. I'm so scared of the side effects."

These statements are a *tiny* sampling of what I hear from my well-intentioned veterinary clients on a daily basis. Many are concerned about side effects from drugs or medical procedures that are invasive. Others are tired of trying to treat a condition with pharmaceuticals that just don't work. More commonly, costly diagnostic and therapeutic procedures are out of range of most household budgets.

The Animals Never Lie is a sampling of successful case reports from my practice where alternative treatments have been incorporated, sometimes alone and other times along with conventional medication. The title was chosen because animals cannot *fake* a response nor do we worry about a *placebo* effect with them. They simply accept natural therapies and innately "know" what is good for them or not. Unlike humans, the animals don't question the natural approach to healing. Therefore, they can't "lie" when a positive change in their condition occurs.

When using a natural product such as an essential oil, it is never *forced* on an animal unless I feel, as its professional caretaker, that it will save a life. The great majority of the time, however, I let the animal "show" me what it needs. I've had dogs try licking lemon essential oil off my hand before I can even get it applied. I've had horses that try to grab a bottle of oil in its mouth while I'm trying to open the cap. My own cats curl up beside my essential oil case whenever possible.

These cases are meant to be a representation of what can occur with the use of safe and effective holistic products and therapies. There are a *lot* of sub-standard or adulterated products out there, so *please* consult with a holistic veterinarian or qualified animal professional before getting on the internet and ordering products. Even some holistic companies have excellent marketing strategies and do a wonderful job of "selling" you on their products, though they may not be able to tell you where the source of their stuff comes from.

The names of the companies whose products I used in the case reports in this book have been intentionally omitted. This book is not to promote a particular brand or manufacturer. *But*, I only use products that have the highest therapeutic benefits, are backed by veterinary research, and have been tried extensively on my own animals first.

For confidentiality reasons, names of clients and animals have been changed. I do personally thank those who have allowed me to use pictures and have given me permission to include their animal's story in this book.

For a listing of holistic veterinarians in your region, you can search on the AHVMA's home page, *www.ahvma.org,* and click on the "Find a Vet" link.

Thank you for taking the time to read this book. Please spread the word that there are other ways to approach your animals' health!

Barbara A. Fox, DVM

Table of Contents

Chapter 1 – Apache

Apache was a sweet fourteen-year-old Paint gelding owned by a good friend and natural horsemanship trainer. Bob called me out to examine Apache, thinking his gentle horse had sustained a back injury. The day before when Bob had tried to mount Apache bareback, the usually gentle and mild-mannered horse nipped him on the calf of his leg. Thinking his belt buckle was digging into Apache's spine, he removed his belt and tried to mount again. This time, Apache sank his teeth into Bob's leg *hard*. Since this behavior was totally out of character, Bob gave him the benefit of the doubt and summoned veterinary help.

Bob had the white and sorrel gelding inside a large steel shed that doubled as an area for hay storage and arena. He had a lead rope loosely draped around Apache's neck. I started my exam by carefully palpating the muscles along each side of the spine. When I got to his lower back, he flinched. I could see his muscles bow downward with light pressure from my fingers. Gently, I repeated the pressure; again, his spine caved downward. Convinced that Apache had strained his back, I intended to apply several essential oils along the sides of his backbone to help with inflammation and pain.

I opened my case of essential oils and removed the bottles I needed for the treatment. However, my eyes kept diverting to an oil blend that was used almost exclusively for digestive support. It contained oils such as fennel, tarragon, peppermint, patchouli, and ginger. Since I had started using alternative methods in my practice, I knew that intuition was something that a person learned to trust. So I opened the bottle and let the horse sniff. He smelled it for a very long time, then attempted to chew it. Not wanting a broken bottle in his mouth, I promptly pulled it away. Apache continued to "look" for it, which was a positive sign he needed the oil blend, for whatever reason.

I went back to collect the oils I had chosen, but again, my eyes fell on frankincense. Frankincense oil has a multitude of uses and activities, so I opened the bottle not knowing why I was drawn to it. I let Apache take a good whiff of it. Within a few seconds, Apache pushed against me, as if intentionally trying to move me out of the way. I put a few drops of frankincense on his jugular veins but before I could step out of the way, Apache shoved against my hip, almost knocking me down. Immediately afterward, the gelding dropped onto the dirt floor and rolled several times. He leaped up, trotted a few feet to a bale of hay, and yanked a few stems of the dried vegetation into his mouth and chewed frantically.

Again, Apache dropped to the ground and rolled five or six times rather violently. By this point, I was nervous that he was having some kind of reaction to the oils. I'd never seen behavior like this and wasn't sure what was making Apache roll. For the second time, the odd activity culminated with a mad dash to the hay bale for another mouthful.

"Bob, I'm quitting with the oils for now. I don't have a clue what's going on and I don't want to cause him any more discomfort."

"Hey, Barb, that's fine. I trust your judgment," he replied. "Maybe we can try it tomorrow. I've never seen him like this before. Sorry he slammed into you."

"I know. This isn't 'Apache.' Why don't you keep an eye on him for the rest of the day and if he's still acting strangely in a few hours, give me a call, okay?"

I never heard back from Bob that evening. Later the next morning, I called to check up on Apache. "Well, you'd think we had an elephant here overnight," Bob reported.

"What are you talking about? An *elephant?*" I didn't understand what he meant.

"I kept Apache in a stall overnight instead of turning him back out in the pasture. This morning when I went to do chores, you couldn't even see the floor. There was so much manure it was unbelievable."

Wow. It suddenly hit me as to what had been going on. Apache had an intestinal blockage, or impaction, causing him to be sore when Bob tried to climb on him. Even though the horse hadn't shown any signs of colic, he was dangerously constipated. I shuddered as I thought of what conventional medication might have done (or not done). Anti-inflammatory meds and painkillers would have been given to treat a suspected back injury, perhaps causing more distress, or possibly causing the impaction to become life-threatening. This horse "knew" what he needed and tried to communicate in the only way he could.

Apache recovered completely from his episode. The next afternoon, Bob took him for a short trail ride without any signs of discomfort or unwillingness to perform. Bob and his wife routinely use essential oils in their training facility, especially after witnessing the profound turnaround in their own horse.

* * * *

Author's note: Animals WILL let you know, sometimes in unorthodox ways, that there is a problem. They don't concoct or embellish stories to gain attention. They are down to earth creatures, living in the present moment. Getting to know one's animal is crucial for their wellbeing, both physical and mental. In my "journey" into holistic practice, animal communication (a.k.a. psychic or intuitive) skills are important to be able to read what the animal is feeling or thinking. Even though you don't have to be a professional communicator or a psychic, you'll have an inner "knowing" that something isn't right.

In my earlier years of veterinary practice, I would have scoffed at the idea of an animal trying to tell me something. I now know differently, and encourage animal owners and other animal professionals to listen to their intuition when it concerns their precious pets and livestock.

Chapter 2 – Chipper

Daschunds are interesting little dogs. Nicknamed "wiener dogs" because of their long body and relatively short legs, they have their own unique physical challenges. Picture a suspension bridge. There are no supporting beams to help hold up the bridge; both sides are simply anchored to the earth. Dachshunds have similar conformation—their backs are long—and there is nothing to support the extra length. As a result, it is not uncommon for these dogs to suffer ruptured spinal discs, especially if they're already overweight.

Such was Chipper's case. He arrived at the mixed animal practice where I was working one Friday afternoon around 1:30 p.m. Chipper had been running through his backyard the day before when he hit a little hole in the ground and fell, severely twisting his back. He was unable to stand or move his rear legs at all.

This type of presentation is a medical emergency. Once disc material protrudes against the sensitive spinal cord, surgery is usually the only way to decompress the nerves. It has to be performed before permanent damage sets in, or the swelling and inflammation moves upward. Respiratory paralysis can result if the condition progresses. In less severe cases, strict cage rest and anti-inflammatory medications can sometimes alleviate the symptoms.

Chipper had *no* sensation in his hind legs and lower back when I examined him. He had been injured twenty-four hours earlier, and I was very concerned that all of his function had been lost. However, if "deep pain" was still present, there was a chance for recovery. I got out a small pair of hemostats and gently pinched the skin between Chipper's toes. He pulled back, which is a normal response, and I was greatly relieved to discover the reflexes to be present. Before I explained treatment options with Tina, Chipper's owner, I made a quick call to one of the neurologists at the state university's veterinary hospital to get a quote for back surgery.

I was quoted $5,000 for surgery alone. The emergency fee, hospitalization, and myelogram would be up to $1,500 extra. The specialist also informed me that we had exactly three hours to get Chipper to the veterinary hospital, since it was a Friday afternoon and there would be no one available after five o'clock. If surgery was withheld another twenty-four hours, I was warned that Chipper would never walk again.

"Tina," I explained carefully, "they need Chipper right away. They're concerned that if you wait, he may be permanently paralyzed." Her chin began to quiver and tears filled her eyes.

"Okay, Dr. Fox, I understand. I just have to ask though. How much are we talking about?"

I discussed the fees with her, carefully outlining what the surgery and aftercare would entail. Several tears rolled down her cheek. Tina hesitated as she reached into her purse for a tissue. "I —I just can't do it. Financially, emotionally—there's no way…" she confided. "I don't have an extra $5,000 sitting around. Money has been tight for us ever since my husband started trade school."

The look of despair was written all over her face. How I felt for her. When a pet's treatment plan exceeds the client's pocketbook, the options are frightening.

"So what do I do? I can't just put him to sleep!" Tina exclaimed.

I took a minute to think about what I could offer her. Tina was already familiar with alternative medicine and energy modalities like Reiki. She was already using essential oils in her own human family. "Tina," I said as I put my hand on her shoulder. "Of course, surgery is the 'Cadillac' treatment for conditions like Chipper's. But I totally understand where you're coming from. Surgery is expensive and you already know there are no guarantees. If you're open to trying some alternative therapies, let's get started."

My client was ready to try anything to help her little furry kid. We decided to incorporate corticosteroid therapy (at my insistence to get him "jump started" in his healing), daily applications of essential oils and massage therapy, homeopathics, and a special diet. Chipper would be hospitalized for several days so I could have my staff carefully monitor his condition. Since he wasn't able to void his bladder or have a bowel movement on his own, we would need to manually express the urine and feces until his nerves began functioning again.

On Day 1, Chipper received a small dose of dexamethasone to help with inflammation and swelling in his spinal cord. He also got essential oils of oregano, thyme, basil, wintergreen, cypress, marjoram, copaiba, and peppermint on his back. The staff administered homeopathic tablets to help with pain control and to promote healing. Chipper seemed to love the attention, especially when we massaged the essential oils onto his neck and back.

The same protocol was repeated for Day 2. Our little canine patient seemed much more alert and was able to hold his upper body steadier. We still had to help him with bathroom duties, but it was still too early in the healing process to expect big improvements.

However, on Day 3, we had some surprises. When my technician arrived at the clinic early to administer morning meds to our patients, she found Chipper *standing*—just for a few seconds—he had regained enough strength in his legs to hold his body! Not wanting to get too optimistic, I told Tina it was a good sign, yet if Chipper was active *too soon,* he could regress and be right back to square one. At this point, I cut out the steroid medications and increased the essential oils treatment to three times daily.

On Day 4, Chipper had urinated and defecated in his cage overnight. Normally, that would cause us to groan, since *no one* wants to face a kennel full of poop and pee first thing in the morning! But my technician and I shared a "high five" because our patient was able to go on his own! Everyone in the clinic was just amazed at the little dog's progress.

On Day 5, our friendly Chipper was standing for short periods of time, although he couldn't yet walk. By this time, I was confident that Tina could take care of Chipper at home. Since she lived a little over two hours away, I set up a recheck exam in four weeks, unless he had a setback. I gave Tina specific instructions on which oils and supplements I wanted her to provide at home, knowing that she would be totally compliant with the recommendations.

* * * *

Four weeks from the day that the university neurologist claimed Chipper would never walk again if emergency surgery wasn't performed, he waddled into the exam room, vigorously wagging his tail. It seemed as if Chipper was expressing his gratitude toward us, and we were elated to witness him walking unassisted. I commended Tina on being diligent with Chipper's therapies, as oftentimes success in healing comes from careful attention to following through with protocol.

Chipper continued to improve, with a minor setback one year later. He had fallen down a few of the basement steps, but with a few days of rest, he was completely back to normal. He lived to the age of fourteen, where he died at home from causes unrelated to intervertebral disc disease.

Chapter 3 –Livestock Truck Rollover

Driving back from an essential oils event on a warm Saturday afternoon in July, I rounded the top of a hill and witnessed emergency vehicles with their intense flashing red and blue lights on the opposite shoulder of the highway. In the westbound ditch, a double-decker livestock semi was laying on its side in tall grass and weeds. I immediately slowed my vehicle to a crawl.

As I approached the scene, one of our local EMTs and volunteer firefighters, Ron, was directing traffic. I rolled my window down to talk with him and then I heard the the pitiful screams of injured, trapped, and dying pigs. The noise made me sick to my stomach. *"Do you need any help!?"* I shouted. My husband Gary was also a firefighter and had lots of experience with hogs, having raised them for years on his family's farm. Since the accident scene was only a few miles from home, Gary could be there in a few short minutes.

"We can use all the help we can! There's a hundred and eighty-five pigs in that trailer," Ron yelled. *"We gotta get 'em out as fast as we can and onto another trailer!"*

I quickly dialed my husband. He'd already heard of the accident over the fire radio and was already en route. In the meantime, volunteers, sheriff's deputies, and emergency workers set up temporary corrals in the ditch and adjacent field to hold the animals. I racked my brain, trying to figure out how *I* could help. I had my entire case of essential oils with me. *How could I utilize them in the best manner? These poor hogs left a confinement facility, were prodded onto a ramp, and forced into a crowded semitrailer.* Not only were they suffering physically, but mentally and emotionally as well.

The first group of two-hundred-and-thirty-pound pigs were extracted from the twisted metal of the trailer. Scraped up, bleeding, and dazed, they stumbled into the makeshift pipe corral. It had been the first daylight the pigs had seen in their lifetime. Scared and hurting, they milled around, knocking into each other. Some were open-mouthed breathing due to their injuries and were in shock. A trailer containing gigantic plastic water tanks was positioned beside the pigs, and workers started spraying the downed animals with cool water since the heat and humidity would eventually take a toll on them.

I grabbed a full bottle of frankincense oil and climbed into the holding pen. Making my way through the group of dazed animals, I sprinkled the oil on their heads, backs, and directly into the mouths of those who were down and suffering. Frankincense essential oil, in my opinion, can be tremendously beneficial for uplifting the spirit and increasing the will to live. The surviving pigs were going directly to the slaughterhouse, but if their quality of life could improve even for a few hours, I felt it was worth it.

A second enclosure was erected for the next batch of survivors. I couldn't get to that pen, so I handed the bottle of frankincense to one of the emergency workers and asked him to sprinkle the oil onto the pigs. The noise from the screaming animals and the equipment used to cut through the metal sides of the trailer made it difficult to hear. The worker gave me a deer-in-the-headlights look. I shouted, "Trust me, I'm a veterinarian—it's a bottle of medicine!"

"Oh, okay," he yelled back as he started liberally peppering the pigs with oil. I wanted to tell him it only took a *few* drops per animal as I watched the pricey oil being doused. But there was no time to talk as more animals were being unloaded. Later, I found out he joked to his buddies that I gave him some "holy stuff" to treat the pigs with. *Whatever,* I thought. If I saved one life today or alleviated suffering, it was totally worth the ridicule.

The very first pig I put frankincense onto had looked pretty bad. He had been down on his side, with multiple scrapes, bruises, and cuts. After twenty minutes, he was standing, yet feeble. Soon afterward, he was rooting in the grass and walking as if he'd never been injured. Hogs raised in confinement never get to see or feel the outdoors, so to witness him pushing his nose along the ground was impressive as well as heartwarming. Several of the other pigs I treated with frankincense were also making a fast comeback.

Others weren't so lucky. Overall, eighty-five animals perished in the accident. Many were crushed to death by the sheer weight of the other pigs toppling onto them. Volunteers worked well into the evening, transporting the survivors back to their original facility and cleaning up debris from the accident.

My husband had a hard time dealing with the sights, smells, and sounds as he had been inside the semitrailer helping to free the trapped animals. No matter how detached you try to be, it's painful to watch any animal suffer. Fortunately, we had another small bottle of frankincense at home. Both of us sniffed from it deeply to help erase the painful memories of the day.

Fortunately, the driver of the tractor-trailer rig escaped unharmed. He apparently had a sneezing fit which caused him to temporarily lose control of the semi, dropping the outer tires onto the shoulder. Those few seconds of unavoidable distraction, however, could have cost him his life as well.

* * * *

Author's note: Never underestimate the power of alternative therapies, especially essential oils, in situations that are far from "routine." Even though these animals were headed for slaughter, their pain and suffering needed to be diminished or eliminated if possible. Some would say, "Well, they're just animals," but they feel pain and experience emotional trauma much the same way as people. In my opinion, all animals deserve compassion and care whenever it can be given.

Chapter 4 – Miracle Kitty

Mid-to-late afternoon is a common time for emergencies to walk in the door of any veterinary clinic, and today ours was no exception. I was working at a mixed animal practice in northeast Iowa when I was warned by our receptionist that a cat with a collar "stuck" in its mouth was on its way. *How weird,* I thought, *can't the owner just pull it out?* I learned through many years of experience, though, that emergencies were rarely routine and sometimes extremely unique. You can picture the scenario in your mind, but what enters the clinic doors may be something totally different.

My veterinary technician ushered a young woman holding a cat wrapped in a bath towel into the exam room. Even though I was still at least 15 feet away, the stench from this cat's mouth was horrendous. *Well, that's not good,* I surmised, *must be infected like crazy. What the heck are people thinking when they let it get this bad,* I grumbled. *Probably be another late night this week.* In a veterinarian's office, there is no such thing as a regular closing time. At least for the staff.

The cat was owned by a mentally challenged middle-aged lady and the young woman was the caretaker for her. The disabled woman's family had purchased a new collar for her kitty a week ago. When the kitty went missing, the caretaker assumed that it had slipped out the door. No one could find it until an unpleasant odor was detected in the owner's spare bedroom. The cat had crawled under the bed and went into hiding for several days. When the caretaker finally discovered the source of the odor, she rushed the kitty to the clinic.

The collar was bright pink with several silver jewels attached to each side. An elastic nylon band designed to hold a small jingle bell to the collar had somehow become wrapped around the cat's lower teeth and jawbone. Apparently the kitty had attempted to paw the collar off over its head, catching the band behind the bottom corner teeth. The poor feline couldn't close its jaws and there was a copious amount of smelly pink saliva staining its entire face and neck. Worse yet, the band had penetrated through the gumline behind the lower teeth and was embedded tightly in new scar tissue. Skin and muscle around the jawbone where the band encircled it had rotted away, and at least an inch of raw bone was exposed on both sides of the face. I was heartbroken because I knew this type of wound with exposed bone would necessitate euthanasia.

"You don't understand, Dr. Fox," the caretaker explained, "you *have* to try to save this kitty. She has been a godsend for my client. Her condition has gotten so much better since she's had her for a companion."

"Oh, that's so sad," I responded, "but here's the situation." I drew a deep breath and concentrated on the reality of the cat's condition. "There is severe infection inside of the mouth and the lower jawbone. Worst case scenario, the bone may die. The cat may completely lose its entire jaw since we don't know how much circulation has been compromised. Teeth may fall out. The infection may have already spread to internal organs, causing them to fail. She can't even close her mouth, so there may be nerve damage to her jaw which we can't fix. If she can't eat or drink on her own, then she'll have to have a feeding tube inserted. She's already quite dehydrated, and putting her under anesthesia is high risk."

"I know, but I plead with you to at least *try.*" Her desperate tone of voice caused me great anguish. I knew the prognosis would be critical, if not grave.

Reluctantly, I put together a treatment plan and a cost estimate— this would be an expensive case—and for what? For the cat to lose its jaw or die from a deep and painful bone infection? Struggling to push my thoughts out of the way and attempting to be objective, I showed the young caretaker the complete list: intravenous fluids, anesthesia, injectable antibiotics, pain medications, debridement and tissue repair, and days of hospitalization. Before I got half way through the treatment schedule, she interrupted me, saying, "The family only has $200.00."

I gazed at her and dejectedly sighed. "That doesn't leave me very much to work with. I don't own the practice and I can't alter the prices without talking with the owners of the clinic first. And please, if the kitty means that much for your client, check with the family and see if they'll allow for any extra funds."

The caretaker quickly called the family and explained the severity of the cat's condition. They agreed to allow another one hundred dollars to be used to treat the kitty. Still, I knew that several days of hospitalization and repeated treatments would be well over the range that had been permitted. The clinic's owners decided to take several payments rather than charging the handicapped client all at once. Relieved, we prepared the cat for surgery.

As we clipped away hair and cleaned the wounds with straight saline, I racked my brain as to how I could treat this cat without spending a fortune. Luckily, the clinic's owner allowed me to purchase essential oils and use them as needed. I knew that if this cat's life was to be saved, essential oils would be my best bet—and the least expensive way to go.

Once the kitty was anesthetized, I carefully excised the elastic band from the gingival tissue and flushed the rotting tissue with a blend of saline water, cinnamon, clove, eucalyptus, rosemary, and lemon essential oils. Then I added helichrysum, copaiba, frankincense, and lavender. They were also applied to the exposed bone and surrounding tissue. Normally, I would have diluted the oils with a carrier oil such as olive or coconut oil, but this cat's life was at stake, so the oils were used full-strength. We carefully cut away decomposing tissue until healthy flesh was seen. A commercially-prepared salve containing essential oils was packed onto the exposed bone. Antibiotic injections were also given, along with intravenous fluids to help rehydrate our patient. Not very optimistic for her survival, we placed the wounded feline in a warm cage and checked her vitals. She seemed to be very stable and comfortable.

When I arrived at the clinic the next morning, I was apprehensive about checking on my patient. I hadn't expected her to live overnight. Jan, my technician, met me in the hallway.

"You're not going to believe what you're going to see," she said solemnly. "Hold onto your hat."

Now I really *was* worried.

As I rounded the corner to the cat ward, I saw a black tiger striped kitty standing in its cage, hungrily devouring a can of prescription food. At first, I wondered if another cat had come in during the evening. Then

I realized that this was the same kitty I'd given a death sentence to just twelve hours earlier!

Amazingly, the kitty improved so well after three more days of essential oil therapy (diluted with a carrier oil for these treatments) and antibiotic injections, I discharged her without any take-home meds. I knew the owner and caretaker wouldn't be able to treat the energetic little feline and I was a little concerned about not continuing treatment past three days. But by this time, healthy new tissue was completely covering the exposed jawbone, and the mouth sores were filling in nicely.

The family was ecstatic, and to this day, our little miracle kitty is still doing very well. Amazingly, the bone healed without infection setting in, which had been my number one concern.

And no more collars for our furry friend...

* * * *

Author's note: Yes, at times, even I am totally shocked at the healing powers the body possesses when it's given a chance to rally. Had I "listened" to the little voices in my head saying 'there's absolutely no hope, forget the family's wishes and put this kitty to sleep,' we never would have known this little feline could pull through. Although I am adamant about never wanting an animal to suffer needless and unresolvable pain and suffering, giving this patient a chance confirmed my decision to see what miracles could occur.

This case was submitted and accepted for publication by the Journal of the American Holistic Veterinary Medical Association.

Chapter 5 – Lacy's Lick Granuloma

One of the most frustrating cases to treat is a dog that incessantly licks one or more of its legs to the point where there is a deep, chronic lesion. The scientific name for this condition is "lick granuloma." No one really knows what causes a dog to develop one, but it's theorized that pain from arthritis or a previous injury, an allergic reaction, or a foreign body (something that penetrates the tissue and is still embedded) causes enough inflammation that the dog licks and chews until a deep wound is created. It's also considered a type of obsessive-compulsive behavior because once the dog starts licking, it cannot or will not stop.

The worst case I'd seen was where a black Lab chewed its left front leg so badly that the tendons were exposed and the bone eventually became infected. That was when I was still in conventional veterinary practice and nothing worked on that poor dog. Eventually, the dog was euthanized because the infection took over the entire foreleg, although the animal had been on several month-long courses of antibiotics.

Lacy, a sweet, 10-year-old yellow Lab, walked into my office along with her owner, Ed. He'd called me a few days prior and asked if there was anything I could do naturally for the lesion on Lacy's front leg. Apparently Ed's regular veterinarian had dispensed two different antibiotics for several weeks and the sore was still there. Fortunately, it wasn't a deep wound at that point, but I knew if the licking continued, it would become much worse. Not knowing whether Ed was "on board" with natural medicine, I went through my usual description of what we would do.

"Ed, I never guarantee that the products and the therapies I use in my office will work. Just like with 'regular' medicine, some things will take care of the problem, and others won't. Each animal, each person, is different. If you're willing to try, I'd love to see Lacy."

"I understand totally. I'm not a big fan of going to the doctor myself."

Ed had a tree farm and was an avid conservationist. He claimed he was a "closet" tree hugger and we both laughed. I liked him immediately, as we had something in common. Northeast Iowa was heavily timbered in places, and too often indiscriminate logging took place, which left the hillsides barren and cluttered with dead branches. There is a difference between harvesting trees in a way that promotes regrowth and beauty, and simply going in and trashing out the forest. We had an interesting discussion about that and I was happy to share my ideas with him.

Ed assured me he would do anything I recommended to get Lacy's leg to heal. So, we discussed diet, if chemicals were used to clean the house, any past traumas (physical or emotional), whether Lacy spent most of her time inside or out, and any recent vaccinations or chemical flea/tick preventatives he used. Luckily, Ed's family used natural products in the house and around Lacy. She was on a good quality dog food and routinely got fresh deer meat and other sources of raw protein.

I mixed a combination of frankincense *(Boswellia carterii)*, helichrysum, and lavender essential oils together in a glass dropper bottle. I showed Ed how to apply the oil blend with the dropper directly onto the lick granuloma. I also dispensed a bottle of probiotics since Lacy had been on antibiotic therapy for such a long time. Anytime an antibiotic is given, the beneficial bacteria in the intestines are destroyed, leading to further healing complications from a compromised immune system. Probiotics are crucial for resupplying the gut with "good" bacteria.

"These oils need to be applied *faithfully* three times a day," I instructed my client. "Is there someone in your home that can do that for her?"

"Oh yes, my daughter Lindsey is home for the summer. She'll be the one taking care of Lacy."

"Okay then, I want to hear back in a week or so from you. I'd love to hear how Lacy is healing."

One week went by with no phone call. Unfortunately, I only had Ed's home phone and no cell number. I left a message on their answering machine, but no one called back.

Two weeks passed, then three and still no word from Ed. One day I saw him fueling his truck at the local convenience store. I quickly pulled in and quizzed him about Lacy's condition.

"Oh, that sore healed up so good you'd never know she had a problem in the first place," Ed smiled. "Wow, thanks for helping her out."

Trying to hide my shock, I answered, "You know, that's great news because those are some of the hardest skin conditions to fix. Great job on keeping up with the protocol."

"Yes, Lindsey loves that dog more than anything. She was really worried about her, so she was very diligent about getting those oils on."

Lacy's dilemma had a very happy ending. I ran into Ed almost a year later, and he told me that the lick granuloma never returned.

I had a very happy client and I was thrilled to hear that the wound was gone forever.

Chapter 6 – Blossom's Lymphoma

Nothing stirs up more fear than a diagnosis of cancer. *Absolutely nothing.* Unfortunately for Leon and Diane Jenkins, their kitty, Blossom, had recently been diagnosed with small cell GI lymphoma, an aggressive cancer of the intestinal tract. My clients had never had children, and Blossom, at age eight years, was their child, their world. They were devastated with the news and were very anxious to find out if there was anything in the realm of alternative treatments they could do for their precious feline child.

Blossom's illness became apparent when she started vomiting after eating. Their former veterinarian assumed, as many would, that Blossom had an intolerance for something in her diet based on her main symptom of throwing up undigested food. He changed Blossom's diet to a prescription dry kibble diet that was formulated for sensitive stomachs, and placed her prophylactically on an antibiotic for one week. This therapy seemed to help as the vomiting episodes decreased dramatically.

A few weeks later, however, the vomiting returned, only this time, Blossom was getting sick several times a day. She had lost a pound of body weight and her activity level was alarmingly diminished. Concerned, Leon and Diane took her back to the veterinary clinic. Their veterinarian performed x-rays of Blossom's abdomen as well as a full range of bloodwork to check her red and white blood cells, as well as all of her organ systems. The radiograph showed a suspicious mass near in the upper quadrant of the abdomen, near the junction of the stomach and the first part of her small intestine. Bloodwork was remarkably normal, so Blossom was scheduled for an endoscopy (inserting a tube with a tiny camera down her esophagus and into her stomach and intestine) to investigate further.

Their veterinarian took a biopsy of the mass after the endoscopy procedure revealed red and irritated intestinal lining. The pathology report from the University of Wisconsin described a malignant cancer (lymphoma) that carried a poor prognosis for survival after six months. And that was *with* chemotherapy. Leon and Diane, devastated by the news, were desperate to try anything to save their beloved Blossom.

They were referred to the University of Wisconsin's veterinary teaching hospital at the urging of their regular veterinarian. The cancer specialist carefully reviewed the pathology report, re-examined Blossom, and formulated a treatment plan. It involved giving an oral chemotherapy tablet, chlorambucil, once every two weeks plus 5 mg of prednisone every day. Every three months, Leon and Diane would take Blossom to the university for recheck appointments and bloodwork.

After the second round of chlorambucil, Blossom's vomiting episodes increased significantly. Diane kept a detailed journal of Blossom's illness and in a short period of time, the vomiting was occurring up to ten times daily. On a particularly bad day, she threw up over twenty times.

Leon and Diane knew their kitty couldn't survive much longer if they kept up the current chemotherapy protocol. Blossom now weighed four pounds less than when she first became sick. Her haircoat became dull and flaky. Clumps of fur fell out spontaneously, apparently generated by the chemo drug. Filled with despair, Leon and Diane began to lose hope.

However, the couple had just started using aromatherapy on themselves, and were curious to find out if there was anything that could benefit Blossom, if only to keep her spirits up. The couple searched online and found me on the American Holistic Veterinary Medical Association's website. They were two hours away, but willing to make the trip to consult with me.

I met Leon, Diane, and their beautiful gray and white Blossom at a mixed-animal clinic where I was employed as the small animal doctor. One look at my clients confirmed their love for their kitty. Their faces appeared pained; their concern was evident as they poured out the entire history of Blossom's illness from start to present. Diane had a detailed daily journal of what Blossom ate or didn't eat; when she had a bowel movement; how many times a day she vomited; her behavior (whether somewhat playful or very lethargic). I suddenly felt pressure build as they put their trust and faith in me to help their furry kid. They were counting on me to "fix" their little feline.

"Well, we have a challenge ahead of us, Diane and Leon," I stated, "and the only thing I can promise you is that I will do everything I can to help Blossom. But inevitably, it will be her will to live and your compliance with what is recommended that will pull her through, if that's possible."

"We understand, Dr. Fox, and we're willing to do anything it takes. We know her prognosis is bad, but if we can keep her comfortable, that's our big goal."

I was relieved to hear them talk about comfort, because in all the years of being in veterinary practice, lymphomas were often aggressive and animals usually didn't survive. In fact, I'd never seen a patient live more than a few years after his or her diagnosis, even with aggressive therapy.

Diane was concerned that the chlorambucil was killing Blossom. "Dr. Fox, I can't begin to think about giving her more of those pills. She gets *so sick* afterward! But I'm afraid she'll die if she *doesn't* get the chemo! What do we do?" I noticed Diane's chin start to quiver and tears fill her eyes.

"Then let's talk." I moved away from the exam table and pulled up a chair facing them. "I am 100% for quality of life, not just keeping an animal alive and suffering because the owner isn't ready to 'let go' just yet. Chemotherapy that causes this type of reaction isn't contributing to your kitty's quality of life. It's actually just the opposite."

"But I don't want her to die, Dr. Fox," Diane cried. "I can't lose her. *I just can't.*"

"I totally understand. Believe me, I *do*. But we also have to think about Blossom's discomfort. She is suffering. That's not fair to *her.*"

Leon cleared his throat and asked, ""What would happen if we stop the chemotherapy? Is there a chance we can use something more natural to help her with the cancer?"

This was the really tough part. I was trained, in veterinary school, to only offer "approved" therapies (drugs, chemo, radiation, surgery). Anything else was taboo. On the same note, I had a patient who was trusted to my care—to make her comfortable and to think "outside the box" and to come up with a holistic approach to her dilemma.

"I'll tell you a little about myself," I offered. "Here's my story." I proceeded to tell Leon and Diane about my own cancer diagnosis; my horrible fear of the side effects from conventional treatment, and how I chose to go the holistic route, without any kind of chemo or radiation. They listened intently.

"So now, here's what I'm going to say. I can't tell you to take Blossom off of the chemo drugs. But I *can* tell you what I'd do if this happened to one of my own kitties."

The couple leaned closer and I continued. "After having gone through a tough decision myself, and knowing exactly what the side effects are of the drugs, I couldn't put any of my animals—or myself—through it. I completely believe in the power of prayer, intention, feeding the body what it needs to sustain and repair itself, herbs, homeopathics, and essential oils to help the body *heal itself.* No ifs, ands, or buts."

Leon and Diane's faces immediately softened. I could sense their relief after hearing me give them my opinion. The couple asked for a few minutes to discuss a decision, so I left the room to start developing a long-term treatment plan.

When I returned a few minutes later, Diane still had reservations about stopping the chemo pills. This is where faith must step in. I reminded her that whatever decision she made, she had to believe it was the best one for her kitty.

"Oh Dr. Fox, I'm so torn! But I can't stand to see her so sick either!" Tears were rolling down her cheeks uncontrollably. Handing her a box of tissues, I put my hand on Leon's shoulder and asked him to share his thoughts.

"I'm convinced that we need to stop the chemo and try the other natural products you mentioned. We're already using essential oils so that isn't anything new to us." He turned toward Diane. "Right honey? We can't let Blossom go on this way anymore."

"I guess so. I'm just so scared," Diane admitted.

"It's okay to be apprehensive when you're making this kind of decision. But try not to let your emotions go wild around Blossom. She needs positive thoughts and love, not doom and gloom," I reminded.

Blossom's new protocol was to wean her off of the prednisone and to stop the chlorambucil at the next interval of treatment. I developed a plan to use frankincense, sandalwood, lavender, and copaiba essential oils directly onto the skin over her stomach area. In addition, I made a combination of oils containing oregano, thyme, basil, peppermint, cypress, and marjoram in an ounce of extra light virgin olive oil. The couple was to apply four drops of this blend two to three times weekly on Blossom's spine. The theory behind this type of oil therapy is that the spinal area "holds" a lot of bacteria, viruses, and fungi (some which are postulated to cause cancer), and by applying essential oils over this area, the body may start to respond positively. I also instructed them to diffuse calming oils such as orange, lemon, lavender, and frankincense in the houses where she spent the most time.

We changed her diet to all-canned; I wanted to have them feed a commercially-prepared raw diet, but Diane wasn't yet agreeable to that. I told her that was fine, but we needed to completely remove the dry kibble. There is too much starch and sugar in the form of grains, potatoes, etc. that cancer loves to feed on. I started their kitty on a supplement that was formulated from raw organ meats so she would get much-needed enzymes for her overall health. I also showed them how to administer a potent antioxidant drink by mouth once daily. I felt that product would boost her energy and provide trace minerals and other micronutrients that her diet may have lacked. Lastly, I added a homeopathic remedy to support Blossom's ailing immune system.

Fortunately, Blossom's guardians used all natural cleaning supplies in their home, and there were no synthetic products to worry about. I've found that eliminating things such as plug-in air fresheners, scented candles, commercial cleaning supplies with harsh scents, etc. can turn an animal's health around once they're away from the chemical assault. This is especially important in cancer or autoimmune diseases where harsh chemicals can play havoc on the body.

Not wanting to shift things too quickly in Blossom, I advised Leon and Diane to start with this protocol. I've had animals that detoxify too quickly and that could cause more harm than good. So we set up an appointment for a month out to see how Blossom responded.

At her four-week checkup, I was very encouraged at her appearance. Blossom's coat was shinier; her eyes were brighter, and she was only vomiting a few times a week. She had gained a pound back and was starting to play on occasion. Cautious not to be overly optimistic, I praised Blossom's guardians for their diligent care and encouraged them to keep up the good work.

The next month's checkup was even better. Blossom looked bright, alert, and happy. Her caretakers reported she was chasing a play mouse, and her appetite was improving each week. By now she had gained another pound, although she was still under her normal weight. I asked Diane how the treatment plan was going.

"Well, I almost had a heart attack one night. I read the directions wrong for mixing up the combination I'm supposed to put on her back."

"Oh no, what happened? What did you do?" I quizzed.

"Instead of putting on just four drops of the mixture, I put the whole ounce on her back! She started drooling, then got really quiet. I thought I was going to lose her."

I quickly calculated the amount of oils this cat received. One ounce of olive oil plus 28 drops of essential oils. Wow! That was a *lot*. "So Diane, what did you do? How did Blossom fare after that?"

"Well, Leon whisked her off to the tub and rinsed her off right away, but the olive oil, geesh, it was so hard to wash off. Her hair looked terrible for several days." Diane appeared embarrassed at her mistake.

"Good to hear you rinsed her off right away. How was she afterward?" I was curious to hear if she had any ill effects from all of the oils.

"Funny thing," Diane mused, "was that she actually felt pretty good the next day. She started running around, like her 'crazy cat' routine thing before she got cancer. I thought we had the 'old' Blossom back again!"

That incident proved to be the turning point in Blossom's health. Although I always caution my clients to use as little essential oil as possible, since they are so powerful, in this case it turned out to be just what this kitty needed. She continued to flourish despite nearly drowning in oils. (I've always said there are no "accidents" in life.)

* * * *

Blossom and her pet parents continued to come to my office

for semi-annual checkups, which were always a joy. By now, Blossom had far surpassed her six-month prognosis, and in all respects, was a healthy, sassy feline. She lived to the age of fourteen and a half, when she suddenly developed liver failure. Leon and Diane declined having an autopsy performed, so it wasn't known if Blossom's cancer suddenly reappeared, if she had a bad batch of food, or a latent virus attacked her liver. She was only sick for a week before her caretakers made the tough decision to have her humanely put to sleep.

Blossom was truly another miracle kitty. She lived almost seven years (in great health) after her initial diagnosis of lymphoma. Had it not been for the meticulous care she received from Diane and Leon, she may have succumbed earlier. It was a great honor to have known this family.

Chapter 7 – Valentine's Behavior Change

Valentine was a beautiful 5-year old Boxer who had suddenly started biting the children and other family members she lived with. I was shocked to hear this, since I had previously treated "Val" at a different veterinary clinic and had absolutely no problems with her. In fact, she was a sweet, docile girl and I always enjoyed seeing her. Today, in my office, she seemed fearful and withdrawn. As she crawled into her caretaker's lap, I heard a low growl. I slowly backed away from Nancy and her anxious girl and pulled up a chair several feet away.

"So Nancy," I began, "tell me more. You said Val started biting your son and his friend. Has she bitten anyone else in your home?"

Val was tightly curled in a ball on Nancy's lap. She eyed me warily.

"Yes, she nipped at my husband and Nate, our adult son." Nancy shifted uneasily in the chair, then told me, "The biting has been more frequent. I'm afraid to have anybody come into our house. My biggest fear is that I'll have to put her down."

"Oh Nancy, I'm sorry to hear this. It's so uncharacteristic of Val! She has always been the sweetest dog in the world. What do you think may have changed her demeanor?"

"I can't pinpoint it, but my husband and I are separating. Our kids aren't dealing with it very well, so I'm sure there's more tension in the house than ever."

I nodded in agreement. "The animals are super sensitive to people's feelings, even if you're trying to 'hide' them," I explained. "They seem to know just what's going on. So what we need to do is dive a little deeper into this emotional situation all of you are sharing."

Nancy shifted uneasily in her chair, then sighed and told me she was leaving her husband and moving in with her female lover. In the twenty-some years she and her husband had been married, Nancy admitted she had been living a lie, and now that everything was out in the open, she felt a big relief. However, the rest of the family was reeling from the confession. No wonder Val was picking up on everyone's negative energy. The poor canine didn't know how to deal with the emotional chaos in the home.

"Nancy, the way I'm going to attempt to help Val is to offer her some essential oils to smell. The theory behind how they work when they're smelled is this: when Val inhales the oils, the aroma will go directly through her nasal receptors inside her nose, then the molecules of oil will enter the bloodstream. From there, they travel quickly to the limbic area of the brain, where hormones and emotions are manufactured and stored. Our goal is to let the essential oils 'do their work' to release the non-beneficial feelings your friend is storing there."

"I'll try anything to get Val to quit biting and attacking. I can't stand the thought of having to put her to sleep."

"I don't want you to do that either, Nancy. I know this little girl is loving and wants to be with you. We need to help her sort out everything that's been happening in her environment. I'm going to offer Val several different oils for her to smell. Are you okay with that?"

Nancy nodded in agreement. I opened a bottle of essential oil that was blended specifically for its peaceful and calming effects, putting a few drops in my hand and offering to let her sniff my palm. Val looked intently at me for a few seconds, then cautiously dropped her nose to my open hand and inhaled with quick, short breaths. Not wanting Val to view me as a threat, I sat cross-legged on the floor in front of Nancy and brought the oils up to Val's nose. Each oil I offered her—including a blend designed to release the "trapped" emotions, one to instill confidence and courage, one simply called "Hope," another to address the "child within," and one to help with adjusting to new situations—was met with curiosity and concern as she eyeballed the bottle with her nostrils fluttering. Within a few minutes, I was able to touch her back as Nancy gently held her head.

I put a few drops of a combination oil that may promote confidence onto Val's back and stroked her softly. Her eyes softened as she turned to see what I was doing. Next, I rubbed a few drops of a blend intended to be stress-relieving on my hands and petted Val with the oils.

No signs of aggression or tension appeared, so I pushed further ahead with the emotional release session.

Reassuring Val that nothing was going to harm her and that she could let go of trying to protect Nancy, I "showed" her a mental picture of what would happen if she continued to bite people. (I've learned from professional animal communicators that animals "talk" in pictures.) Using the oil blend called Hope, I applied this to the top of her head, along with a few drops of frankincense and told her what a beautiful, loving girl she was. At this point, Val crawled down from Nancy's chair, curled up in my lap, and licked me on the cheek! To say the least, I was amazed and totally shocked. I hugged Val and let her know I was so proud of her change.

Two weeks later, Nancy called to say Val hadn't attempted to bite at all and was warming up to the two sons again. I cautioned Nancy to continue with the oils I'd sent home with her because I wasn't convinced Val was truly over her issues yet. But the behavior never resurfaced. Val was finally "free."

* * * *

Author's notes: *Family conflicts and an unsettled environment are just two reasons for animals' "misbehavior." Animals are very sensitive to negativity, tension, and anger amongst their humans, creating an unhappy and stressed environment for all.*

Although there are animals who are born with certain aggressive tendencies, most of the detrimental behavioral issues (such as cats not using the litter box) can be traced to an imbalanced home. Most animals require a "safe" room or space where they can retreat to when chaos ensues. Providing your pets with as quiet and calming of an environment as possible is very important to their mental and emotional state.

Chapter 8 – Jack's Digestive Issues

I believe we have it all "wrong" when it comes to medicine, whether human or veterinary medicine. Having had cancer and choosing to forego conventional chemotherapy and radiation, and instead turning to products from nature to bring balance and support back to my immune system, I see a huge problem with how we view our doctors' limited recommendations (surgery and drugs). Now of course, there are naturopathic and integrative physicians who understand that our traditional medical model falls short (or is over-emphasized) in this culture, and I commend them for their open minds and faith in the natural process of healing.

Too many times (and this is a gross understatement), I see patients on the brink of death. Their guardians have trusted in the conventional medical model, much to their dismay when it fails. They do their research and find that there are "alternative" products such as western and eastern herbs, homeopathics, essential oils, acupuncture and chiropractic, flower essence remedies, sympathetic resonance light devices, biofeedback products, etc... but instead of *starting* with those modalities, they put their trust in their traditionally-trained doctors and veterinarians and listen to conventional recommendations. Now their beloved animal friend is terminal or suffering greatly and they want help. Unfortunately, it's oftentimes much too late.

I believe that beginning therapy with alternative medicine is the only sensible way to go, *provided* the animal's condition is *not* acute (meaning sudden onset) and conventional medication is needed to save its life. The good majority of the cases I see in my office are chronic in nature, such as allergic dermatitis, auto-immune conditions, heart failure, and cancers. These are usually conditions that have been "smoldering" for a while. So steroids, antibiotics, diuretics, and drugs that suppress the immune system are prescribed, further deteriorating the animal's body. Sometimes these drugs are needed; however, I am adamant about supporting the body's various organ systems with a diet that is close as possible to its natural food requirements, whole food supplements, essential oils, homeopathics, and a healthy emotional state, *then* resorting to pharmaceuticals if all else fails.

A good friend of mine adopted a Jack Russell terrier from her local humane society. "Jack" was a happy, healthy, energetic little guy. Why he was relinquished to the humane society, no one seemed to know. His owner, a well-intentioned pet owner, fed her dogs a highly renowned, somewhat expensive dry dog food, thinking she was feeding a quality product.

After several months, Jack developed bouts of intermittent vomiting and loose stools. The episodes occurred infrequently and only lasted a few days. After Jack recovered from them, he seemed perky and playful again. It really bothered Annette, though, worried her little guy was suffering from a serious disease.

Even though Annette and I had been friends for a good many years, she was not sold on alternative medicine. She chose to consult with her regular veterinarian, who ordered all of the pertinent blood tests, abdominal x-rays, fecal exams, and a thorough examination. All of the results came back normal, except for very mild elevations in Jack's liver enzymes. With little to go on, the veterinarian started Jack on an antibiotic, thinking he may have had a mild bacterial enteritis (intestinal infection). Jack recovered uneventfully but a month later, had another episode.

This time the vet added metronidazole, which is another antibiotic used for intestinal upset. He also prescribed an acid reducer, thinking Jack might be suffering from acid reflux. Again, Jack recovered quickly. However, a third bout that occurred just three weeks later had Annette even more worried.

Jack's veterinarian rechecked Jack's liver enzymes, and again, they were slightly elevated. Jack was prescribed Science Diet I/D, a bland prescription canned food that is used to settle the intestinal tract down while an animal recovers. He put Jack back on another round of antibiotics just in case he hadn't completely recovered from his previous "infection."

Annette was becoming concerned, because her spunky little terrier was becoming thinner and his haircoat appeared dry and dull. At her insistence, Jack's doctor referred them to Iowa State University's veterinary hospital for a full workup with clinicians who specialized in internal medicine. Jack received ultrasounds, digital xrays, additional bloodwork to rule out a primary liver problem, but nothing out of the ordinary was discovered. After paying her bill, which amounted to nearly $3,000, Jack and Annette drove home with no prescriptions, no special food, or any future recommendations.

When Annette told me about her experience at the teaching college, I got firm with her. I told her I wished she'd consulted with me first, before spending an extraordinary amount of money to come up without a diagnosis or advice on how to stop the intestinal upsets. "What would you have done differently?" she asked, puzzled.

"Well, first of all, I'd get Jack off of the dry kibble food. I don't care *how* expensive it is or how many testimonials this food gets. Get him on a raw diet, or if you're not comfortable with that, at least get him on a lightly cooked homemade diet that's formulated by a veterinary nutritionist."

My dear friend admitted she had heard too many negative things about raw diets and was very leery of the thought of "that kind of food." She did, however, start cooking Jack his own meals, using a recipe she found online. I warned her to make absolutely sure she was using a veterinary-supported recipe since there were too many imbalanced diets to choose from. I also suggested two whole food, powdered supplements for intestinal and liver support that she could mix right into the soft food. I also advised her to start a good quality probiotic twice daily. Also, I mentioned placing a drop of two of an essential oil blend intended for overall intestinal support on Jack's belly daily.

Surprisingly, Annette heeded the advice. In just a little over three months, Jack had gained two pounds and his fur had become soft and shiny. The most astonishing—well to her, but not to me!—thing was there were *no more* occurrences of vomiting and diarrhea. Just by getting Jack onto a food without fillers, by-products, artificial flavorings, dyes, and preservatives plus adding micronutrients and probiotics, this little dog flourished.

This is a classic case where starting with *good quality,*

appropriate food and adding nutritional supplements that support the liver and intestinal tract was all the "medicine" this patient needed. I applauded Annette for trusting me enough to temporarily let go of her attachment to conventional medicine and using what nature provided for his healing.

Please teach yourself to read a food label and what the ingredients are composed of. There are *so* many animals that are fed a "good" diet, or so the owner thinks, only to have chronic health issues from the food. Recurring ear infections, skin allergies /itchiness, colitis, liver issues, etc. can often be remedied by changing to a different diet, especially a commercially-prepared raw diet. At least know that grains are genetically modified to the point that the body cannot recognize them, and that pesticides and herbicides from the grain can wreak havoc in the body. They're toxins! Also, meat by-products are anything *but* healthy; they're the rendered parts of the animal, not muscle meat. Growth hormones, estrogen-like products, and antibiotic residues can be found in beef and pork. Chicken and turkey feed have coccidiostats (for parasite control) in them. Fish in canned or dry food may contain high levels of mercury and possibly other heavy metals.

Let's look at a very popular adult maintenance dog food. Here's the ingredient list with a description of each following:

Chicken, whole grain wheat, cracked pearled barley, whole grain sorghum, whole grain corn, corn gluten meal, chicken meal, pork fat, chicken liver flavor, dried beet pulp, soybean oil, lactic acid, flaxseed, (an array of vitamins), oat fiber, taurine, mixed tocopherols, natural flavors, apples, broccoli, carrots, cranberries, green peas.

First of all, the ingredients on a label are listed in order of weight. It might look like chicken is the main protein source, but *chicken* is weighed with the water and fat still attached to it. Once you remove the water and fat, chicken may be 4th or 5th on the ingredient list. On the flip side, *chicken meal* is the product *after* those two things are taken out, so chicken meal would be the preferred first ingredient.

But look at the next several things: wheat, barley, sorghum, corn. These are fillers. Wheat is *the most* genetically modified grain on the planet. Lots of humans have what they think is a gluten insensitivity, when actually they're not able to tolerate the GMO's (genetically-modified organisms) in the wheat. Barley is actually beneficial, and is usually added as a good fiber source. But it's still a grain and possibly genetically modified as well. Then whole grain corn….usually added as a cheap protein source, even though it's hard to digest, not to speak of its high level of modification, toxic levels of pesticides, fungicides, and herbicides. Sorghum is another inexpensive source of protein, but again, it's a grain, with potentially the same risks with genetic alterations and pesticides. Corn gluten meal would carry a risk for gluten intolerance. Dried beet pulp is often sweetened with molasses or syrup, adding calories and increasing the carbohydrate load. Soybean oil is better than soybean meal, although here we go again: it's a widely modified (genetically) product. The rest of the ingredients appear to be good, although flaxseed is very unstable in heat, and kibbles are processed under heat pressure. That means that your pet will be getting almost zero benefits from flaxseed in the dry food.

Lesser quality foods contain even *more* undesirable components, such as BHT (a toxic preservative), red, blue, and yellow dyes which can be considered allergens or toxins (by the way, dyes are a marketing technique for the consumer. *The animal could care less what color his food is!*) Also included in really cheap foods are meat and bone meal (source of animal protein is unknown and may include several species), more by-products, and chemical preservatives.

* * * *

Author's note: *The message I want you to take home is this: many medical conditions can be cleaned up with a good diet, proper supplementation, and essential oils for overall body system maintenance. Before you go directly to the doctor for yourself—or your veterinarian for your animals—seek natural therapies first. You can always resort to conventional medication if need be.*

Chapter 9 – Vaccine Aftermath

I was asked to do a house call for a large beagle that had developed a severe neurological disorder. The eleven-year-old male exhibited significant head and neck tremors and his head tilted awkwardly to one side. The poor guy could not stand for more than a few seconds before his rear legs, being weak and uncoordinated, couldn't hold his body up any longer. The symptoms started gradually, then become progressively worse over a three-week period. Amazingly, his appetite was normal as well as his bathroom habits. He simply had to have help standing to urinate and pass feces.

The young couple who had adopted Max had initially rushed him to their veterinarian, where the standard treatment of steroid therapy and antibiotics were prescribed. The drugs had little effect on Max, and his condition progressively declined. The veterinarian referred them to the University of Wisconsin's Veterinary Medical Teaching Hospital, where a full battery of tests, including a myelogram and CAT scan were performed. The only thing that the scan showed was a small amount of swelling near the base of the cerebellum. No tumors, cysts, or any other lesions were found. Max was given more anti-inflammatory therapy and discharged with instructions to follow up if his condition didn't improve by the time the medications were done.

Max's female owner, Lana, was just learning about holistic medicine and called me to see what might help her beloved canine. I told her, as I tell all of my clients, that I would strive to find out why Max *had* these odd symptoms, then formulate a plan that could help his body rebalance itself. I told her there were no guarantees but I would do everything in my power to help.

When I first saw Max, his head and neck continuously shook. The constant tremors caused the muscles on both sides of his neck to be tight with multiple "knots". He patiently lay on their couch, padded with a large fleece blanket, while I palpated his neck and back. Except for the rigid muscles, nothing out of the ordinary was discovered.

Because Max was a "foodie," he cooperated well when I offered him a treat to see how flexible his neck was. Though it was difficult for him to remain steady when turning his head, he readily moved it to receive his tasty morsel of food. Next, I needed to have Max stand up to assess his proprioception. Proprioception is a sense of the relative position of the body, or in other words, how the body "knows" when it's in the "right" position. It also can be used as an indicator of the animal's equilibrium.

Lana held Max up while I picked up his left rear foot and turned it under. A normal response would be for the dog to flip it back in its regular position immediately. Max couldn't "tell" where his foot was and made no attempt to correct his stance. He wobbled and swayed, then fell on his side with a big grunt.

His whole neurological assessment and test results from the university perplexed me. I suggested chiropractor care, but the owners assured me they'd already tried that. There had been no change in Max's condition. I quizzed them about acupuncture but there were no veterinary acupuncturists within several hours of their home.

I decided to use a technique called "Raindrop," where a certain sequence of oils are placed onto the spine in several places. The theory behind the technique is that many organisms, toxins, and/or viruses may reside in the spinal column, where the immune system has a harder time working. The molecules of oil are tiny enough to penetrate almost any tissue in the body, including what scientists call the "blood-brain" barrier, so when oils are applied on top of the spine, the oils are close to where they need to be absorbed.

Max acted apprehensive when I brought out the essential oils. I let him sniff the bottle first (as I do with any animal patient) and then dripped a few drops of the oil onto his back. I gently feather-stroked the oils through his fur. Pretty soon, Max relaxed and rested his head between his two front paws. I repeated the procedure with eight other oils. By the time I was done, his eyes were partly closed and the tremors had miraculously stopped.

Max was also started on a homeopathic remedy used frequently for trauma and injury as well as one for pain. We decided on two whole-food supplements for immune and nervous system support. His diet was already homemade and well balanced, so I didn't change anything.

The young couple again asked me what I thought was causing Max's unusual symptoms. I told them I really had no clue, so we went through Max's history meticulously from the beginning. Heart worm preventatives, flea or tick products, chemical exposure in the home—these questions had to be asked. Still, there was nothing that had been given chemically and the young couple cleaned with all natural products. Then the question that triggered my conclusion: when was Max last vaccinated?

The woman thought for a minute, then she said, "He just got his shots about two weeks before this all began."

"What vaccines did he get?" I asked, quickly attempting to put pieces of the puzzle together.

"Well, he got all of them."

"Can you show me your paperwork, Lana? I would really like to know what Max got for his shots," I pried.

Lana had Max's records neatly arranged in a manilla folder. She handed me the latest invoice showing the inoculations he received: distemper, parvo, parainfluenza, adenovirus (all in a combo vaccine), the four-way leptospirosis vaccination, Lyme, kennel cough, and rabies. My mind raced as I felt my blood pressure rising. *Eleven components, all given in the same day. Oh boy, I need to approach this subject carefully. I don't have anything to base my opinion on except exclusion. And I don't want this couple to feel any kind of guilt if my theory is correct.*

"Lana, where were the injections given?"

She pointed to the sides of Max's neck. "He got them all here. Why are you asking, Dr. Fox?"

"You may not be aware of this, but some animals react to their vaccinations. The reaction can occur soon afterward; sometimes later. There is a condition called 'vaccinosis,' which is a hypothetical reaction of an animal's body to vaccines that occurs without the typical hypersensitivity reaction. It can occur weeks or months after the vaccination and can affect almost any organ system. I'm concerned that Max's atypical nervous system problem may have been caused by his last round of vaccines."

"Why haven't I heard of it before? That really scares me!" Lana exclaimed.

"That's because usually only holistic doctors acknowledge this type of disease state," I answered. "Vaccine manufacturers will tell the doctors their vaccines are 'safe', and veterinarians are *not* required to report any suspicious vaccine reaction. You have to remember that vaccine producers are 'in it' for the money, just as any big business. I know, it's not right, but that's what conventional veterinarians bought into, thinking that vaccines are without risk. I was there at one time too! We were told that if an animal had a mild reaction, it was actually *good,* because it meant that the immune system was gearing up to build a great immune response. But that's so far from the truth, Lana." I took a deep breath and continued.

"For about ten to fourteen days after immunization, the immune system is somewhat suppressed. After that period, the immune system goes into overdrive, where it's overstimulated. That's where a lot of autoimmune diseases start. To add insult to injury, there are components in the vaccine like thimerasol, which is a cousin to mercury, aluminum, other animal proteins, antibiotics, and even some traces of formaldehyde. The list could be up to twenty ingredients long! So if you pet has a reaction to a vaccine, it could be to *any* or several of these components."

"Oh, my gosh, I had no idea," Lana said softly. "Is Max going to be okay?"

"I can only hope that the products we chose to use on him will help. Again, Lana, this is only my opinion, but the correlation of his symptoms and his vaccine history are too close for my comfort. Especially since the university couldn't come up with anything from all the tests they ran."

Max made a slight improvement in his mobility and the tremors lessened, but despite aggressive therapy with holistic treatments as well as conventional medications, Max never fully recovered. He lived another year until his condition deteriorated to the point he had to be put to sleep.

Do I believe the vaccines could have created this disease state? Yes. Can it be proven? *No.* Until science comes up with ways of tracking and studying these potentially life-shortening reactions, we must go on the process of excluding any other possibilities. Unfortunately, research may never be undertaken. Why? *To protect the vaccine manufacturing companies' interests.* That's the number one reason.

* * * *

Author's notes: Before you blindly accept your veterinarian's recommendations for what vaccines your animal needs, do your research. Find out what your dog's risk for exposure to things like Lyme disease, kennel cough, canine influenza, or leptospirosis actually is. If your cat is indoors, why be coerced into vaccinating it for feline leukemia? Or yearly distemper combination shots? Vaccines are not a "one size fits all" product. They should be chosen with your animal's best interests in mind.

One final word: if your pet is suffering from any chronic disease, such as diabetes, heart failure, cancer, allergies, or any autoimmune disease, it should not be vaccinated. The insert on every vaccine label clearly states that a vaccine should only be given to healthy animals. Unfortunately, many boarding and grooming facilities require proof of immunization before your pet can come in. Check with your state's requirements for mandatory vaccinations before you book your appointment. Some kennels require kennel cough and canine influenza, at their request, not the law's.

For more information, you can check out recommended vaccination protocols on the American Animal Hospital Association (AAHA) website. They have a link you can follow to find out what you should vaccinate for and how often.

Furthermore, titers can be performed with a simple blood test. A "titer" is a way to check for antibodies circulating within the animal's body against a particular disease, such as rabies or distemper. If the titer indicates that there is indeed protection with an adequate titer level, your animal may not need vaccinated against that particular condition.

Chapter 10 – Scamper

_____

I cringed when I saw Scamper enter the exam room. He was a small but very overweight Miniature Pinscher /chihuahua cross. The poor little guy was carrying his right rear leg up in the air, unable to put any weight on it. I had seen Scamper for the past couple of years for routine checkups and he had never been lame.

"How long has he been this sore on the leg?" I asked Jen, his owner. "Did this start recently or has he been limping for some time?"

"Just yesterday afternoon. Jim saw him running with our other two dogs. When Scamper turned quickly, he stumbled and was limping pretty badly. It's just today that he won't put any weight on the leg."

I gently manipulated Scamper's leg and palpated the sides of the stifle ("knee") joint, checking for swelling or pain. When I extended the leg forward, putting pressure on the ligaments, Scamper winced and pulled away.

"Jen, what I think we have going on is a partially torn cruciate ligament. It's an injury similar to what a lot of football players suffer from. I can't be certain, but I'd venture to guess that's what's going on. I'm not an orthopedic specialist, and to get an exact diagnosis, I'd like to refer Scamper."

"Oh, I can't do that, Dr. Fox," Jen replied, visibly concerned. "Jim just got laid off from work and I'm afraid money is going to be tight. Is there something else we can do that's not too expensive?"

I gazed at the plump seven-year-old dog. I wasn't very optimistic for the knee to heal since he was carrying so much extra weight around. "Jen, I'll lay it straight out to you. You _have_ to get some weight off of him, because there's no way, even _with_ surgery, that the joint will heal. I can put Scamper on some natural anti-inflammatory products and give you a blend of essential oils that will help control pain. The biggest suggestion I have is to cut back on his food."

Jen petted her little dog and sighed. "Okay, I can cut back on his food and treats. Whatever it takes to help my little guy". She leaned over and kissed the top of Scamper's head.

We also decided to use essential oils that would support the musculo-skeletal system, such as balsam fir, blue spruce, lemongrass, wintergreen, copaiba, peppermint, and eucalyptus. Jen was instructed to apply them, diluted appropriately, directly onto the strained stifle joint three times a day. I also sent her home on a homeopathic remedy for pain and inflammation.

In just a little over three weeks, Scamper was walking very well on his injured limb, though he was still slightly *off* at times. Jen had done a wonderful job of limiting Scamper's portions of food, as he had lost one whole pound. On a dog with a small build, one pound looks like twenty! I commended Jen on doing a great job.

Scamper never had another issue with that leg. He lived to be a ripe old age of fourteen.

* * * *

Author's note: Here is an example of why offering natural, holistic treatment is so important when money is a concern. Too many veterinarians will simply say, "Well, there's nothing more to be done. He'll eventually tear or rupture the ligaments of the other leg. You might as well put him 'down' now to save him pain and anguish."

Is that really the only way to look at a case? I shudder to think of the animals that have been euthanized because holistic treatment was never offered, nor was referral to a holistic doctor ever considered. Scamper was given a chance to persevere and against certain odds, he rallied and lived with quality of life until it was his time to pass.

Chapter 11 – The Bull

It was a very busy day in the mixed animal clinic. The morning started off with a male cat who had a severe urinary blockage. It took the better part of two hours to relieve the "sand" and mucus that was plugging the outflow from his bladder. Then a dog who had a bad reaction to an over-the-counter flea and tick preventative presented in liver failure and had to be started on an I.V. Next, a dog who had recently been neutered developed a nasty infection at the incision site had to be admitted to the hospital for intravenous antibiotics and monitoring. And I still had a full schedule of regular appointments.

At this particular clinic, I was the primary small animal doctor, with the other two doctors taking large animal calls and helping with small animal appointments when necessary. Dr. J was in the large animal treatment area trimming hooves on several high quality, expensive Angus bulls. When finished, Dr. J offered to help with appointments so we could get caught up. I heard him tell the receptionist to call Ed and tell him, "If that bull isn't up by morning, we'll put him down."

"What happened?" I asked, curious to know what went wrong with a foot trim.

Dr. J confided, "Well, that last bull fought the head gate pretty good as we were cranking up its foot. He went down pretty hard on his front end. Gave him some pain killers but it's not looking good."

Gosh, I hated to hear that. Darn large animal work. It's dangerous not only for the handlers, but the animals too. "What are you thinking, Dr. J? Broken neck?"

"Not sure. Doesn't seem to be a fractured leg, but he might have dislocated a shoulder. Or screwed up something in his back. Ed's coming back soon to pick up the other bulls. I opened up the chute so his injured bull can get into the holding pen. If he's not up by morning, we're going to give him the pink juice."

"Pink juice" was our nickname for euthanasia solution. The liquid is dyed a bright pink so there is no way to confuse it with another injectable drug. Dr. J's nonchalant attitude toward the bull upset me just a little bit. Or to be honest, maybe a *lot*. He knew exactly how essential oils worked wonders on some of the most difficult cases. Last spring, Dr. J was vaccinating a herd of cattle for brucellosis when one of the cows slammed into him, knocking the stainless steel syringe, with needle fully exposed, directly into the top of his foot. The needle penetrated his rubber boot, shoe, and sock, with the tip buried in his foot. Brucellosis is a bacterium which causes abortions in cattle. Since the vaccine (RB51) is a modified live vaccine, it can cause "undulant disease" in humans when it enters the body. There was enough vaccine on the tip of the needle that stuck in Dr J's foot to cause it to swell up and start to turn black overnight. The seasoned veterinarian knew enough to start on antibiotics immediately, which did help him from getting sicker, but the pain and swelling was immense. I had him apply balsam fir, clove, peppermint, wintergreen, helichrysum, and lavender essential oils to the foot three times a day. Within just a few hours, Dr. J felt better and was getting some relief from the pain. Combined with the antibiotics, Dr. J was able to keep working despite his infected foot. He fared better than most humans with the disease; in rare cases it can be fatal. The healing time was incredibly fast, with no ill effects.

"Dr. J, would you consider letting me try some oils on that bull?" I begged. "You've seen firsthand what they can do. It can't possibly hurt to try."

The middle-aged veterinarian sighed, then crossed his arms and smiled at me with a look of, "Whatever," written on his face. "You're just going to waste those oils, but if it makes you feel better, go ahead. At least the treatment area will smell good," he chuckled. Ignoring his smug expression, I walked away, determined to prove the power of the oils.

After all of the small animal appointments were over with for the day, I checked on the bull. He had struggled enough to get himself out of the chute and was laying up against the rails of the holding pen. Perfect. I wanted to get the oils directly onto the back of his neck and sprinkle them all the way down to the base of his tail. First of all, I let him smell an oil blend that was affectionately called "chiropractor in a bottle." I figured that would be my foundation oil; one that would help that spine align itself before I started applying the rest. He inhaled deeply. I was cautious to not get too close to his head, because one huge swing of it against my arm could break it or dislocate a shoulder. Bulls are never to be taken for granted; even the most docile-appearing animals may turn on a person without warning.

Jan, the receptionist, joined me in the back area to watch me work on the bull. I immediately put her to work uncapping bottles of oil and handing them to me as I asked for them. We used oregano, thyme, basil, peppermint, wintergreen, copaiba, marjoram, cypress, and helichrysum on the back. Since the massive bovine was leaning slightly our direction, I simply dripped the oils onto the fur and carefully feather-stroked them in toward the skin. Before I had the last oil on his spine, the bull rolled straight onto his chest and attempted to rise. He only got a few inches off of the ground, but at least it was an attempt.

Dr. J had already gone home. The pressure was off to try and explain my rationale for doing the oil therapy. Jan was more open than anyone else in the clinic to alternative medicine, as she had seen Dr. M and Dr. K perform miracles with essential oils, homeopathy, and acupuncture. Those two doctors were no longer with the clinic, but Jan's eyes had been opened after having witnessed miraculous turnarounds.

I figured I had nothing to lose by trying the oils. If the bull *did* manage to get up, he would live. If he *couldn't* make it up, he would die. It was unfathomable to me to not try to save his life. Using only my fingers that were saturated with oils, I tapped along the allegedly affected area of the spine for several seconds. It was an "energy" technique I'd learned from Dr. M.

One more strong application of the oils was made before I locked up the clinic and headed for home. I prayed for a miracle.

Bright and early the next morning, I noticed the large animal treatment area was empty. Concerned that the bull had died overnight and his body had already been moved, I cornered Dr. J.

"I see Ed's bull didn't make it. Sorry for that loss."

Dr. J looked at me funny. "Well, whatever *stuff* you put on him last night must have worked. He was standing up and eating this morning. Ed already came and got him."

I stood there, speechless. Even though I *knew* about the power of essential oils, I hadn't really held out much hope for the injured bull. The odds seemed too slim for any kind of decent recovery.

* * * *

There is never any case that is too bizarre, too serious, or too insignificant to try alternative therapies on. You never know when you might save a life.

Chapter 12 – Sophie's Mass

Essential oils were something I was still becoming acquainted with when Sophie arrived at my office one bright Thursday morning. Her owner, Kendra, wanted me to look at a growth on one of Sophie's toes. She'd already made an appointment to have the mass removed at another veterinary clinic, but Kendra wanted a second opinion before subjecting her dog to anesthesia and surgery.

Sophie was an attractive, middle-aged, female Chesapeake Bay Retriever. I watched her as she walked around the carpeted lobby of my office, checking for any signs of lameness, which might help me determine if the mass was invading sensitive nerves or other structures.

Fortunately, she didn't favor the foot. Sophie shyly climbed onto the chair beside Kendra. I palpated the round, hairless lump that was situated on top of her toe. It felt partially attached to the underlying tissue. The mass was slightly irregular, with a reddish tinge around the margins. I didn't like to see these types of growths, because oftentimes they were malignant. Luckily, the lymph nodes in her armpit were normal-sized, and the rest of her physical examination was within normal limits. I could sense the apprehension in Kendra's voice as she asked me what I thought it was.

"I can't tell you if it's cancerous or not. Only a biopsy or taking it off and sending it in to a laboratory for histopathology are the only ways you'll know for sure," I replied cautiously. "I *do* know that the veterinarian you're seeing for removal of the lump will take off the entire toe, not just the mass. He'll want to make absolutely sure, if it is cancerous, that he doesn't leave anything behind."

Kendra stroked Sophie's neck, deep in thought. "What would you do, if this was your dog?" she timidly asked.

I cringed. I disliked this question more than *any* other. It's not that I didn't like giving someone my opinion; it's just that almost everyone goes along with what *I* would do for my *own* animal. It must be an individual decision—for that animal in question *only*—based on the animal's best interest *and* the financial situation of the client, as well as the animal's comfort and quality of life.

"Kendra, I can't speak for Sophie, *but* if it was *my* dog, I'll tell you my honest opinion."

She leaned forward and nodded her head, anxious for my answer.

"You have to know my story, having had cancer and going totally holistic with my approach to getting well. I truly believe that trying to remedy a health issue with natural products *first,* and resorting to medical intervention later, or in conjunction with natural therapies, is the only logical way to proceed."

I waited for my client to process the information. "What products would you suggest?" she asked.

"For starters, we would rely heavily on essential oils such as frankincense to help reduce the tumor size. There's been a lot of research on boswellic acids, one of the most important constituents in frankincense oil, in causing tumor cells to die without compromising the healthy cells. There are nutritional supplements that can promote a healthy immune system, which is needed to get this mass under control. After a few weeks, let's evaluate the lump, and if we need to tweak the protocol, we can do so at that time. Also, if you are worried about cancer and want to have the growth removed, then you should keep your appointment with Dr. Johnson."

"I'm already familiar with essential oils since my sister started using them several years ago. I just don't know how to use them in animals yet." She shifted on her chair, sighed, and then stated, "I won't be taking Sophie in for surgery. I'd like to try a holistic approach first."

"No problem, Kendra, I'll help you get started." I mixed up a combination of oils including *Boswellia carterii*, lavender, helichrysum, tsuga, myrrh, and sandalwood. Kendra was instructed to apply the oils three times daily, then she would bring Sophie back for a recheck exam in a few weeks. I started her on two whole food supplements to support the gastrointestinal tract and liver, key organ systems for toxin removal and excretion.

In just a few weeks, the mass was only half of its original size.

There had been some swelling and oozing from the lump, which is a normal effect of the oils working to kill the unwanted cells. Once the lesion dried up, healthy tissue replaced the shrinking tumor. In a few more weeks, the entire mass was obliterated. Both Kendra and I were shocked, yet elated. Even though I had faith that the products we chose to treat her lump with would do their job, there is always a curtain of uncertainty, depending on how the animal responds.

Fortunately, Sophie's mass never returned.

Chapter 13 – Molly's Itch

Karen was a new client that was searching for ways to alleviate her little Shitzu's extremely itchy skin. Her regular veterinarian had diagnosed Molly with allergic dermatitis, prescribing the typical treatment of prednisone and antibiotics. Prednisone is used to suppress the immune system, which stops the itching. Antibiotics clear up any infections that result from raw and broken skin when the animal scratches. As I always teach my clients, *allergies are a multi-factorial problem. Steroids (prednisone) and antibiotics do NOTHING to cure allergies; they are only band-aids to treat the symptoms.*

Molly didn't do well on the prescription medications, developing loose stools and becoming lethargic. Once the meds were done, the itchiness came back just as bad as in the beginning. Karen confided she had taken sleeping pills the last two nights, since Molly's incessant scratching kept her awake.

When they arrived, Karen grabbed two overflowing plastic shopping bags out of the back seat of her SUV, juggling them and the little white and grey dog. I remember telling Karen to bring any supplements or other natural products she had currently been using. Little did I know it would be bags full!

"I brought all of the things I'm giving Molly now," Karen exclaimed. "I want you to look at them and tell me what you think," she said breathlessly as she shoved them at me while Molly circled excitedly, wrapping her bright pink leash around her owner's legs.

"Let me help you," I offered, fearful she would lose her balance from her legs being tethered together. Grabbing the bags and pushing a chair toward my client, I had Karen sit down and start filling out a new patient form. Fortunately, she had also brought along the medical records from her regular veterinarian. It was evident that Molly had been seen for skin issues for several years. She was on a prescription dry kibble diet for skin issues, along with prednisone and her third round of antibiotics in the past two months.

Karen handed me the completed patient form and anxiously awaited my opinion. She was a concerned, well-intentioned pet owner and I wanted to take time with her and explain what we were going to change in order to help Molly. My first mission was to make sure she knew that holistic medicine may or may not clear up an issue, just as "regular" medicine is never guaranteed to work the way we want. Karen nodded her head in agreement.

"I totally understand that, Dr. Fox," she said, "and I know it will take time. It's not an overnight fix." Karen was well-informed and quite open-minded, making my job much easier.

I examined Molly's skin, carefully lifting tufts of fur to check for flea dirt, inflamed skin, and other abnormalities. Her skin was a bright pink color and felt warm to the touch. She had lost fur on her hindquarters and on all four feet, where she had been biting and chewing. Taking a sample of skin cells and placing them onto a microscope slide, I examined them carefully for evidence of mites, yeast spores, fungal elements, and bacteria. Not finding anything out of the ordinary, I agreed with the diagnosis of allergic dermatitis.

"Karen," I said hesitantly, "let's talk about Molly's diet. I see you're feeding her one of the recommended foods for allergies. I'm going to be completely honest with you—I'm not a fan of these diets at all."

Karen interjected, "Why not? It's expensive and it says it's for skin issues. I thought I was giving my little girl exactly what I should be." Not wanting to accidentally offend her, I started my explanation carefully.

"I totally get where you're coming from, Karen. When I was in vet school, we were always told this company's food was the best you could buy. Little has changed over the years, since the big pet food manufacturers fund many of our continuing education classes as well and almost of the colleges' nutrition courses. Of course, your veterinarian is going to advise that food for Molly since he doesn't know any differently."

I continued, "Holistic doctors study nutrition in depth; it's something we were never exposed to in vet school, with the exception of a couple of hours of the basics. We were never told that all health begins in the gut, meaning that there are the largest number of lymph tissues and nodes in the intestinal tract. So if the digestive system isn't 'fed' correctly, toxins, bacteria, and chemicals damage the lining of the intestines and the animal (or person) will develop what we call 'leaky gut syndrome.' This, in turn, causes those 'invaders' to leak out into the space around the organs. The body recognizes these things as something foreign and sets up an inflammatory response to push them out of the body the fastest way possible. This is the main basis for skin allergies. The body is trying to purge this stuff out, and since the skin is the largest organ in the body, it takes the brunt of the assault."

Karen sat quietly, processing the information. After a few moments, she asked, "So, what is in the food I'm giving Molly that would be harmful to her digestive system?"

"That's a good question, Karen. Let's look at the label." She had brought along an empty bag of the food. "First of all, we want to have a meat source as the first ingredient, *not* grain. All ingredients are listed in order of weight, so having a meat source as the first thing on the list is very important. What's the first on your label?"

"Oh geesh, it's corn starch."

"Okay, is that something you want to give Molly for the main ingredient in her food?" I quizzed.

"Oh no, of course not!" she replied emphatically.

"So read me the next three ingredients," I requested.

"Hydrolyzed chicken liver, powdered cellulose, soybean oil…" I could tell Karen was catching on quickly. "I've never read a label— I'm shocked at what's in this food!"

"I understand. The majority of pet owners never look at the components in the food, or maybe they don't understand what a proper label should include. Let's look at corn starch, the first thing on the label. It's actually considered corn flour, and is most often used as a thickening agent for sauces, gravies, and soups in the human kitchen. It's derived from the endosperm in the middle of a corn kernel. To get to the endosperm, the kernels are processed so all the shell is removed. It's a carbohydrate source *only;* there's no protein, fat, vitamins, or minerals. You know, when people are told to reduce the amount of processed foods in their diet, we never really think about stuff like cornstarch. It's in a *lot* of products."

"Let's move onto hydrolyzed chicken liver," I urged. "The process of hydrolysis uses chemicals to break down the chicken liver to get to the important amino acids. But it's also processed at high temperatures, which kills important enzymes. Basically, you're left with something with very little nutritional value. The third ingredient, soybean oil, is often preserved with BHA, a potential cancer causer, as well as propyl gallate, another possible carcinogen and intestinal tract irritant. Do I need to go on?"

Karen disgustingly responded, "I can't *believe* foods like this can even be sold!"

"I know, neither can I. But with the advent of genetically-modified foods, which we are told are perfectly safe, it doesn't surprise me at all anymore. Cheap additives in our food supply are commonplace and won't go away soon. Now that I mentioned GMO's, let me tell you that with all the modified organisms being spliced into DNA, there is no way the body can 'recognize' these things, which is going to lead to more allergic and autoimmune conditions."

"So what do I feed Molly?" I could feel the concern in Karen's voice.

"You need to start Molly on a commercially-prepared raw diet, or consult with a veterinary nutritionist who can formulate a homemade raw diet for you."

"I've heard that raw diets are full of bacteria and might cause more harm than good. So you're telling me that's false too?"

"Karen, our animals' systems were designed to accept a heavier bacterial load than ours. A raw diet provides all of the necessary enzymes, vitamins, minerals, and other micronutrients that our animals need. Of course, if you're going to prepare your own homemade raw pet food, you'll want to watch where you purchase your meat source. Obviously stay away from large discount chains. There are a lot of local farmers that maybe aren't certified organic but they don't use antibiotics or hormones in their livestock. Just stay away from the factory-farmed meats."

Karen agreed to start with a commercially-prepared raw diet that she could purchase online and have it shipped directly to her house.

Then she handed me the overflowing bags of supplements, asking me for my opinion.

"Here's my take on all of these products. I don't use or recommend anything that is not backed by research, is not veterinarian-approved, or doesn't have a technical veterinarian on staff to answer my questions. There are so many products on the internet that I don't have a clue as to what is actually in them. They're *not* regulated, so there's always a chance that more harm than good can be done."

I was on a roll. "In addition, Karen, you're giving *so* many things to Molly, how would you know if she's sensitive to one of them? Did you consider that you can actually create an *imbalance* in her nutrition if there are too many vitamins/minerals being given together? If I were you, I'd stop giving each and every one of these products at this time. Let's formulate a new plan."

Molly would receive two whole-food supplements for her liver health (which almost always is an issue with allergies, regardless if the liver blood tests come back normal) and one for support of her immune system. These would come from a company who grows their own organic plants, only sells to licensed medical practitioners, and has several veterinarians on staff to take inquiries and make recommendations. She would also be getting one drop of copaiba essential oil orally each day for inflammation. To support her digestive tract, we would start Molly on a pinch of a highly-potent probiotic with nine live strains of beneficial bacteria, as well as digestive enzymes to help her break down the proteins in her diet. Topically, Karen would apply oils such as lavender, frankincense, melaleuca (tea tree), with liquid coconut oil to her fur twice daily. Diffusers throughout the house would help keep a consistent level of essential oils in the air, relieving stress for everyone in the home.

After just a week, my client called and was elated that Molly's scratching episodes had diminished greatly. Within a month of starting on the new diet and supplements we had agreed upon, Molly was pretty much itch free. Karen was extremely happy with the results, and became an avid advocate of natural therapies for both her pets and her family.

* * * *

Author's notes: *Far too many times, diet is never discussed when an animal suffers from systemic allergies or sensitivities. For both animals and people, what you put into your body must be analyzed before starting with a treatment protocol. The importance of feeding an animal what is biologically appropriate is grossly underestimated in the conventional medical office. Scare tactics from large, powerful commercial pet food companies work well to suppress information containing the benefits of homemade and /or raw diets. Consumers are told that the risk of salmonella will kill or sicken their animals, but like I mentioned earlier, animals have been eating meat from their prey for thousands of years. In my opinion, there is much more chance of illness or death from tainted commercial pet foods.*

For more information, I encourage you to check out Dr. Jodie Gruenstern's book, Live with Your Pet in Mind, *available on Amazon and at Life Science Publishing. Dr. Jodie has devoted a significant section of the book to feeding a raw diet and how to properly interpret a food label. She is a holistic veterinarian in Scottsdale, AZ.*

Chapter 14 – "Mighty Mike"

My husband and I live on a rented acreage in northeast Iowa, where we are surrounded on three sides by steep hills and timber and an expansive field of hay on the other. Wildlife is abundant, with deer, wild turkeys, coyotes, and bald eagles frequently seen or heard. Occasionally, there is a screech owl scolding a possible predator or the more hair-raising scream of a distant bobcat. Unfortunately, we had an overabundance of raccoons who were not welcome on the property, as the "masked" bandits would climb over the wall of the feed room, creating a disastrous mess of everything.

There were also feral (wild) cats living in another building when we first moved to the rented acreage. Over the years, Blackie, the "alpha" female, eventually became tame enough to not run away from us every time we looked at her. Her primary joy in life was raising kittens. Although we had no tomcat hanging around our place, she sought out the attention of a neighboring male. She loved her babies, and as her trust in us grew, she paraded her kittens proudly in front of us. But because of the variety of wildlife that like the taste of feline flesh, not too many of her offspring made it to adulthood. Those that did survive were neutered or spayed and given appropriate veterinary care provided we could catch or trap them.

Last spring, two feral females gave birth to kittens which were originally healthy and robust. The mommas brought their kittens up to the house and made "nests" for them in the thick day lilies and plume grass lining the foundation. One of the kittens, a bold, grey tiger striped female, warmed up to me as soon as her eyes were open. As she got older, "Cammie" was the social butterfly of the kittens, always playing and mingling with her siblings and cousins. Even when engaged in serious play time, Cammie would bound toward me as fast as her little legs would carry her if she noticed me from a distance. Her brother and best buddy, Winston, was a cute little tan male; the two of them went exploring together and were pretty much inseparable.

Somehow, after thirteen years of having a very healthy cat population, illness set in. Several kittens stopped nursing, lost weight, and faded away. Most of the adults were not affected, but a few of them developed loose stools and went off their regular appetite for a few days. I couldn't figure out where the sickness came in, or what it actually was, although it appeared to be feline panleukopenia (distemper). We had not had any new cats on the property for the past several years. I did my research and found that raccoons can carry feline distemper virus, which was news to me, since I thought only dogs could contract distemper from coons…at least that's what'd learned in veterinary school. We had a female and three of her young ones trying to steal food from the outdoor cats about a month prior to this outbreak, so this seemed to be the only logical way the distemper virus was introduced to the cats with the exception of an asymptomatic "carrier" in our cat population.

One by one, kittens faded and were never seen again. Winston became ill, but despite trying to force fluids and food on him, he eventually crawled off somewhere and presumably died. I was scared to death for Cammie's health, but the bold little kitten stayed healthy. I'd mixed up some essential oils to support the immune system, highly diluted with olive oil, and placed a tiny bit on the lymph nodes under her jaw, as well as on the kittens that were tame and catchable. I did this procedure three times a day.

One morning, I saw a pathetic little tan kitten fading away in the same manner Winston left us. I picked up his terribly scrawny body and was shocked when he started fighting the restraint, as he seemed so weak. This little guy had a lot of energy for his tiny little body. I put out a teaspoon of canned food, which he half-heartedly picked at. He was dehydrated, so I mixed a few drops of a nutrient-rich juice made from essential oils and wolfberries with a few milliliters of water and syringed it into his mouth. I also placed diluted essential oils on his lymph nodes, to support his immune system.

The next day, my little tan friend seemed perkier and was eating on his own. I felt confident we were past the worst. However, I didn't see him for almost twenty-four hours, when he finally reappeared. I gasped at how emaciated he was; every bone in his frail little body was visible. The moms, who co-mothered all of the remaining kittens, ignored the failing kitten. The only other feline that wanted anything to do with him was Cammie. She licked and rubbed on the little guy's face, as if trying to increase his will to live. I was just about ready to give up and put him humanely to sleep, but suddenly he meowed and tried feebly to climb onto my tennis shoe. I picked him up again and he started purring. This little guy was *not* ready to give up!

Gary and I decided that the sick kitty needed to be in the house, out of the cool morning and evening air, and in Cammie's comforting presence. Since our indoor kitties had their series of vaccinations as kittens, I wasn't overly worried about spreading disease. Cammie claimed a fleece kitty bed I'd purchased a few days prior, and our little tan kitty collapsed beside her after his liquid meals of water, canned kitten food, and wolfberry juice. He was about the same age as Cammie but only half her size. She curled around him, keeping her warm tummy next to him as they both napped.

"Gary, what should we name this little guy?" I asked.

"Tiny?" he laughed. "There's not much to him at all. I've never seen such a skinny animal, ever."

"Okay, find another name. Some day he won't be so 'tiny.'"

Gary was eager to name our survivor kitten as I'd always named the others. Now it was his chance. "How about 'Mikey?' We can call him 'Mighty Mike.'"

"Hey, I love it! Mighty Mike it is!"

Over the course of the next few weeks, it was difficult finding something Mikey would eat. The only thing that *really* tripped his trigger was organic pork liver. We'd ordered half of a pig from a farmer that used essential oils in his livestock and who took as natural and holistic of an approach as possible. His pork was very delicious and I trusted that the organ meats were as pure as I could find.

After I cut a portion of the liver into tiny slices, I held the tiny little guy in one hand, offering him a sliver of liver in my other. He just about took my finger off with the slice of pork! His eyes widened dramatically as he sniffed frantically for another piece of the tantalizing meat. I was elated to find something he liked. For the next week, Mikey ate slivers of raw liver, a few drops of raw egg yolk, and NutriCal, a high-powered, nutrient-dense gel made for animals who needed extra nutrition. He got his essential oils daily too.

Slowly, Mikey gained weight. One by one, his bones became invisible as good, healthy muscle covered them. Cammie continued her vigil of watching over her little buddy, even encouraging him to play with her favorite toy mouse.

Over the course of six weeks, Mikey became a healthy, strong, and playful kitty. His purr vibrated so loudly that we nicknamed him "Rattle-box." Our little tan kitty is now a vibrant, happy one-year old feline who still loves his raw liver.

Chapter 15 – Sadie's Cruciate Tear

Sadie, a sweet, mixed, large-breed dog, injured her back and her right rear leg after chasing a stray cat through the back yard. Limping pitifully, she hobbled to the bottom step of her owners' deck and guided by her own innate intelligence, stopped and waited for help. Her guardian, Rick, had watched his charming girl stumble and ran across the wooden deck to assist. Groaning slightly, he wrapped his arms around Sadie's lower abdomen, clasping his hands together, and lifted the seventy-five-pound dog's rear legs off the ground as Sadie clambered up the steps using her front end. This was the second time Sadie had injured herself in the past few years. Usually rest and anti-inflammatory medications had "fixed" the problem. Yet Sadie was showing signs of chronic joint disease which was very concerning to Rick and his wife, Paula.

I'd seen Sadie for checkups for the past four years. The right rear leg had been slightly uncomfortable at her first visit, which we attributed to past trauma (abuse) she had endured before her present owners rescued her. Today, she resisted full flexion of her stifle and hip joint. When I extended the leg forward, she turned around and tried to snap at me. Knowing this was very uncharacteristic of her naturally mild demeanor, I was highly suspicious of an anterior cruciate ligament injury. The cruciate ligament helps stabilize the stifle ("knee" joint), and a torn cruciate ligament is unfortunately not uncommon in large breed dogs. When I was in veterinary school two and a half decades ago, the injury wasn't seen often like it is today. Many theories exist as to why the cruciate becomes weakened enough to tear, including genetics, dietary imbalances, exercise that is too strenuous, etc. My own personal belief is that the overly-processed modern dry diet is lacking in vital nutrients for good musculoskeletal health, especially when larger dogs like Sadie don't get adequate exercise to keep the soft tissues of the joints strong and elastic. Prior injury can also weaken the tissue to the point where it is more prone to trauma.

Surgery is the preferred option (and usually the only one discussed) in a conventional veterinary practice. Pain relievers and anti-inflammatory drugs are often prescribed before surgery to repair the torn ligament, although they only treat symptoms of discomfort and do nothing to heal the tissue. Sometimes surgery works; sometimes it doesn't. To top it off, the "good" leg is more prone to injury as it has to bear additional weight that the bad leg cannot. Bilateral cruciate tears become a real possibility.

Rick and Paula were nervous at the mention of surgery. Although I knew they probably wouldn't go for the "Cadillac" treatment, I had to mention it. If a veterinarian doesn't give all conventional options, he or she is in danger of being sued. (Although a doctor is never in risk of litigation for not mentioning holistic/natural therapies.)

"I just can't see putting her through this at her age," Rick said. "If there's a chance she won't be any better, there's no way I'd do that to her."

Paula nodded in agreement. "What else can we do, Dr. Fox? If we don't do surgery, tell us what might help her."

I sat down across from Rick and Paula with a note pad in hand. "I'll be very upfront with both of you. I would still encourage you to see an orthopedic specialist, to make absolutely sure that the cruciate is the only thing going on here. The orthopedic doctor will sedate Sadie, take digital x-rays, and perform a detailed exam of the leg. Then, if you wish to decline their treatment recommendations, we can talk."

"I'm going to tell you right now, Dr. Fox, we most likely will not take Sadie to the specialty clinic. I don't want to put her through that stress, but if there's something you can help us with to make our girl more comfy, I'm all for that." Rick leaned back in his chair and folded his arms across his chest. "I hope you don't think we're bad pet owners; it's just that I know my dog and I'll do anything for her except to put her in the car for a three-hour drive because I know she will freak out."

I had to agree with Rick, as I knew how anxious Sadie got during car rides. I usually made house calls so she didn't have to endure a dreaded ride to my office.

I documented my client's decline for referral, for obvious legal reasons.

"Rick and Paula, you know why I have to mention the referral option. Since you've decided how you want to proceed with Sadie, let's get started."

We discussed diet, which was already good but could be improved with the addition of whole food supplements that were designed for musculoskeletal and endocrine support. Secondly, I performed an essential oil treatment on Sadie's spine, using oils of wintergreen, peppermint, blue spruce, lemongrass, vetiver, and copaiba. To keep her relaxed and calm, I made them a combination of orange, lavender, lemon, valerian, vetiver, and Roman chamomile. Leftover mix was left with them, with instructions to apply the oil combo twice daily. Since Rick and Paula already were familiar with essential oils, I told them which oils to keep on hand for extended therapy. Sadie's injury would take time to mend itself. Thirdly, a homeopathic remedy for trauma and pain was prescribed. Last, but not least, I gave the number of a trusted veterinary acupuncturist and chiropractor to them.

Rick offered to design a ramp so Sadie didn't have to navigate steps until healing was complete. He and his wife also agreed to use a beach towel under Sadie's belly to "sling" her when she had to potty, taking the stress off of her injured leg and Rick's tender back muscles.

In little over a month, Sadie returned to full function of her leg, without drugs, medication, or surgery. Between the oils, supplements, and homeopathics, the senior dog thrived, growing out a new haircoat and looking younger than many of her companions of the same age.

* * * *

Author's notes: *Very few cruciate ligament injury patients are ever given the option of trying anything except surgery. Not only is surgery expensive, aftercare is lengthy, with the possibility of injuring the opposite leg during the recovery period. Furthermore, surgery is no guarantee that the ligament won't break down in the future, necessitating another procedure.*

If mainstream medicine would simply look at other possibilities for pet owners who 1) may not be able to afford an expensive procedure 2) are fearful of surgery on their older animal 3) want to try something less invasive, we would perhaps have a healthier, more vibrant pet population, and happier pet guardians.

Chapter 16 – Lucy's Heartworm Reversal

If you have dogs, you're probably quite familiar with heartworm disease. Anywhere there are mosquitoes, there is a chance that your dog can be infected with the spaghetti-shaped blood parasite, *Dirofilaria immitis*. The microscopic microfilariae (infective larvae) is transmitted to your dog when a mosquito carrying the larvae bites her. For whatever reason, the larvae have an affinity for major vessels of the heart and lungs, where they live and grow over the next six months to become adult heartworms, reaching several inches in length. Left unchecked, heartworms can grow and reproduce, causing major damage to vessels, lung tissue, and the heart itself. Dogs can develop heart failure, chronic lung issues, and/or experience sudden death.

Lucy, an exuberant, beautiful female black Labrador, was adopted from a Labrador rescue organization in Louisiana and brought to Iowa in March of 2012. Lucy had tested negative for heartworm infestation in February, before leaving the shelter, and again tested negative when arriving in Iowa. Lucy's guardian, Lynette, started her on a commercial monthly heartworm preventative at that time, and continued it year round.

In February of 2013, Lucy had a yearly wellness checkup, along with a rabies booster and her yearly heartworm test. This time, her blood test came up *positive* for adult heartworms. Lynette was shocked, as was the attending veterinarian. The concerned doctor examined a sample of Lucy's blood under the microscope, finding no trace of the infective larvae. At least the heartworm preventative was doing its job. But when x-rays were taken of Lucy's heart and lungs, there was visible enlargement in one of the top chambers of the heart, as well as a significantly widened pulmonary artery. There was no other explanation for the positive tests (two more tests were sent off to different laboratories for confirmation) other than that Lucy must have had heart worms already reproducing in her heart and vessels before she left the shelter in Louisiana.

Conventional treatment for heartworm disease involves injecting an arsenic-containing compound (melarsomine) deep into the muscles along the spine; two treatments twenty-four hours apart are recommended. If a dog has advanced disease, the treatment is not recommended unless the worms are surgically removed from the vena cava (large vein carrying blood back to the heart). The surgery carries a high risk for complications and is only performed as a last resort. Side effects from melarsomine administration include pain, swelling, tenderness at the injection sites, coughing, fever, lethargy, lack of appetite, depression, lung congestion, and vomiting. Less common effects are excessive drooling, panting, diarrhea, coughing up blood, abnormal heart rhythms, and *death*.

Lynette was frightened and appalled at the same time when her veterinarian explained the procedure and possible side effects. In addition, as the heartworms die off, the patient must be kept confined (usually in a cage or kennel) for up to three weeks to keep the heart's workload to a minimum. Too much activity can cause the worms to cause a blockage in the heart's vessels as they die. Lynette knew her overactive Lab couldn't be kept quiet for that long.

Lucy's guardian did her research and found that there was a protocol for a "slow kill," meaning that products other than the dreaded melarsomine could be used to slowly and gradually eradicate the worms setting up "house" in Lucy's heart. Doxycycline, an antibiotic used for a multitude of conditions, has been shown scientifically to kill a parasite *(Wolbachia)* that lives inside of the adult heartworm. The antibiotic also tends to render the female heartworm sterile so it cannot reproduce. Coupled with weekly doses of ivermectin (Heartgard) long term, the parasites die slowly and eventually are eradicated from the body. Lynette opted to start with the slow-kill method until she could decide exactly what she wanted to do.

"Dr. Fox," Lynette said excitedly on the line. "I have a black Lab that tested positive for heart worm disease. I'm scared—no, really frightened—after I heard the side effects of Immiticide. I'm looking at doing the 'slow kill' method of getting rid of Lucy's heartworms. Are you familiar with this?"

"Hello, Lynette. I've heard of it but haven't had a client ask about it. Where did you get my name?"

"I looked you up on the American Holistic Veterinary Medical Association's website. I didn't realize you were so close!" Lynette lived in a city an hour and a half away from my office. I was thrilled to hear someone think that distance was *close*.

" Well, Lynette, if you're looking at using natural products and therapies to get rid of your Lab's heartworm burden, I can definitely help you. I will tell you, though, that there are absolutely no guarantees that what I recommend will do the trick. On the other hand, I can't guarantee that injections of an arsenic compound into her spinal muscles will be effective either."

"Oh, I know, Dr. Fox," my new client responded. "I am adamant about not doing the regular treatment on Lucy. It scares me way too much!"

I continued to quiz Lynette about Lucy's condition—was she coughing, showing signs of exercise intolerance, wheezing—but Lucy wasn't showing any symptoms at all. The only evidence was her positive blood tests and radiographic evidence of heart chamber and pulmonary vessel enlargement. We set up an initial consultation to get Lucy started on a safe and solid protocol.

Lynette was cautioned that it could take *months* before we'd know if Lucy's body was responding to the nutritional, herbal, and energetic support it would receive. Nutritional supplements containing ingredients such as hawthorn berries, wolfberries, omega fatty acids, CoQ10, digestive enzymes, and citrus extracts/essential oils containing high levels of d-limonene (a potent anti-inflammatory) were chosen. Another nutritional product designed to control parasites was also prescribed. Essential oils of helichrysum, clove, thyme, orange, lemon, grapefruit, copaiba, wintergreen, ylang ylang, wintergreen, and ocotea were used topically and aromatically.

I explained to Lynette that these products were not being used to *kill* the heartworms; instead, they were to support the various organs, especially the immune system, so the body could make it unfriendly enough that the worms couldn't survive. The products I chose also could help the body restore and repair itself.

Other the next few months, Lucy accepted the treatment very well, and Lynette did an outstanding job in being compliant with the recommendations. After four months of the protocol, Lucy was blood tested. Lynette was just slightly disappointed when the test still came back positive. I reassured my client that it was pretty early; keep up the same protocol and see what transpired in another few months.

Six months into the protocol, Lucy was *still* heartworm positive, although the little blue test dot was a lighter color. Perhaps we were gaining ground. I decided to ramp up the essential oil administration, adding several more immune-supportive oils to be applied to Lucy's spine. The only "side effect" was that Lucy was even more energetic, literally bouncing off the walls. Lynette and I laughed at the puppy-like bursts of running, as she obviously felt fantastic despite her "condition."

Nine months after starting the "alternative" protocol, Lucy had a completely *negative* test. No more adult heartworms were present. None. Lynette even had another test performed to make absolutely sure she was free of the parasites.

Of course, Lynette was ecstatic at the outcome. And so was I! (We're not sure if Lynette's veterinarian was, because she was pretty adamant that Lucy would die without conventional therapy.) However, I'm always looking to prove that when the body is supported with the "things" it needs to heal itself, it can do so.

Chapter 17 – Cat's Torn Tendon

Cat, a beautiful sorrel quarter horse mare, ruptured the peroneus tertius tendon in her left rear leg, causing much concern and worry for her owner, Kelly. The sixteen-year-old mare had been confined to her stall for the past four weeks, with controlled hand-walking for five minutes daily. Kelly, a dedicated small animal veterinarian, wanted my opinion if there was anything she could do besides to wait and see if it would heal. Kelly had performed cold laser treatments on Cat and had started her on a few homeopathic remedies which seemed to be helping, but the advice Kelly got from two specialists at different veterinary university teaching hospitals haunted her.

"Both specialists told me that I'd have to confine Cat for six months, and even with that, they told me I'd never be able to trail ride her again. The only thing she might be 'good' for is a broodmare. IF she heals enough," Kelly exclaimed when I first met her again after many years. She and my daughter had been good friends in high school, and I didn't know what career path Kelly had taken until she contacted me. I recalled how much Kelly loved this mare—Kelly acquired her as a yearling—and had dedicated all her energy and free time to make Cat her treasured 4H project. They had been a true team.

I cringed at the diagnosis Cat had been given. The peroneus tertius muscle and tendon are a major part of the supporting structure of the hock (a major joint in the hind leg). They are responsible for flexing the hock, and when they're injured, the horse cannot bend the lower part of the leg correctly, resulting in severe lameness. Oftentimes, horses with this type of injury are euthanized as it sometimes takes up to a year to heal—if it *does* heal.

"Oh Kelly, I know how much Cat means to you! Let's work

together to formulate a treatment plan, okay? Unless you're thinking of taking her to the University of Kansas for surgery."

"No surgery. I can't imagine trying to haul her that far with her injury. Besides, there's no guarantee that she'll even be useful as a broodmare if she did have the repairs done."

"I hear you. First of all, I'm going to give Cat a good exam and see what might have caused the issue in the first place." Torn tendons in this location are usually from an overextension of the hock joint, but the tendinous tissue is very strong and doesn't readily tear or rupture unless there is major trauma, such as falling into a hole, or a previous weakness in the area.

The tendon rupture was blatantly obvious when I picked up the hind leg. The stifle (large joint above the hock and in front of the hip) flexes as well as the hock when the leg is lifted off the ground. Both bend simultaneously; there is no other way the leg can move. It was an eerie sight to view this leg in this unnatural position, with the stifle bent and the hock joint straight, making the lower leg stick straight out behind the body.

Next, I focused on Cat's neck since she had been holding it lower than normal. Three areas in her neck were sore when I put mild to moderate pressure on the muscles along the cervical spine. Now what came before, the cart or the horse? In other words, was the neck tender as a result of the injury, or was the painful neck a cause for weakness situated lower along the lumbar spinal pathways? In addition, the mare flinched when my fingers pressed her on the vertebrae in her lower back. The spinous processes were quite prominent, giving her lower back a slightly humped appearance when it should have been level. The condition in layman's terms is "roach back."

"So Kelly, when you saddle her up, does she kind of hold her breath?" I inquired. "Or try to crow hop when you first mount?"

"Once in a while, she'll round up her back and refuse to move when I first get on," Kelly offered, "but she's never tried to buck."

"Well, let's remember to check your how your saddle fits before I leave. It's amazing how many seemingly minor fitting issues can affect a horse's spine." I relayed to Kelly how difficult it was to find a dressage saddle for one of my Arabian geldings, Tysheyn, due to his unusually high set neck and slight dip in his back.

I brought out my SRT light (SRT is short for sympathetic resonance light, which is a device I commonly use in practice) and my case of essential oils. Sympathetic resonance is based on the same premise as tuning forks—the vibrational frequencies resonate with the body—to bring about a healing environment to the injured area. The lights are created using quantum physics principles and cannot be felt physically, although they are very powerful pieces of equipment.

Kelly was not too familiar with essential oils, so I taught her which oils would be helpful, and how to apply them herself. We also talked about the therapeutic value of good-quality essential oils, as I didn't want her purchasing oils that had been chemically diluted or adulterated in any way. I chose balsam fir, blue spruce, palo santo, helichrysum, lemongrass, peppermint, and marjoram to apply to the lower back and neck. I then placed the hand-held SRT device over the affected vertebrae for ten to fifteen minutes. Cat seemed to love the therapy, dropping her head and closing her eyes. I then made a blend of essential oils to place directly on the torn tendon as many times a day as Kelly could manage.

"Kelly, I'm going to have to be honest here. I really disagree with the advice to keep Cat stalled so much. As she heals, she really needs to move, but it has to be very controlled. Is it possible to find a small pen outdoors so she can see the other horses and get some sunshine and fresh air? I still want you to hand walk her at least twice a day — but in straight lines only. When you turn her, be sure to make very wide arcs to avoid stressing that leg." It had never made sense to me to confine an extremity with a soft tissue injury for that long, as connective tissue (tendons, ligaments, muscles) must get good circulation in order to heal. When a horse stands in one place too long, the blood pools in the lower leg and proper fluid exchange in the veins and lymphatics never occurs. Laminitis (founder) is more of a threat when a horse is idle as well.

"Sure, I have a tiny lot just outside her stall. I can put her out in the morning and bring her in at noon. Plus walk her twice a day. I like the idea of having her in sight of the other horses because she tends to get stressed when she can't see them," Kelly replied.

"Great, Kelly, I'm glad you can do that. Miss Cat needs all the help she can get."

To address the emotional trauma behind Cat's injury, I left a few samples of frankincense, along with several blends that were designed to help release the negative feelings associated with trauma. It's postulated that cellular memory is an important factor in healing, and oftentimes emotions are "trapped" in the cells. Where essential oils may be very helpful is in the way they help reprogram the cells after an accident or any kind of physical or mental assault. Horses, being "flight" or "prey" animals, are in a constant state of awareness of physical danger, and are likely to suffer more mental stress than species that are predatory in nature.

In addition to essential oils, SRT light therapy, cold laser treatments, and some conventional pain medications, I started Cat on two different homeopathic remedies for pain and inflammation. I promised to check back with Kelly periodically as to how her mare was healing.

Two weeks later, Cat was remarkably better, and the dimpling just below her hock, where the tendon had ruptured, wasn't visible anymore. Kelly was elated at her lovely mare's progress. I praised my colleague for her diligence and compliance. She laughed, as we both knew from experience in our respective practices that owners didn't always follow instructions.

Just eight months later, Kelly and Cat went on their first "unofficial" trail ride a few miles from their home. Kelly was careful to limit their ride to flat paths with walking only. Over the next few years, Cat healed completely, allowing Kelly to travel with her to some natural horsemanship clinics out of state and to resume their normal trail riding weekends.

Chapter 18 – Managing Gracie's Mammary Cancer

I first met Gracie, a feisty tri-colored terrier, in July of 2013. Her owner, Donald, was an organic feed salesman who raised his own certified organic beef, pork, and chicken. He valued the holistic approach to medicine, especially after he was in a terrible automobile accident a year prior to our first appointment. Suffering a major head injury, his physician recommended he check into a long-term care facility, as the doctor was very concerned about Donald's lack of balance, short-term memory loss, and lingering effects of the brain bleed he'd suffered. Donald hated hospitals, and the thought of being in a nursing facility both frightened and angered him to no end. He demanded that the doctor release him from his care immediately. His adamant and stubborn attitude paid off, as the doctor reluctantly let him go. Donald then sought out a naturopathic doctor out of state (as Iowa doesn't allow naturopathic doctors to practice), making a three-hour trip several times a month for almost a year to receive the treatments that made sense to him. He made an amazing recovery, with Gracie at his side at the entire time.

Donald ended up "firing" his conventionally-trained veterinarian after she wouldn't see Gracie unless her vaccinations were updated. Angry at her mandate, Donald brought his vivacious little twelve-year-old dog to me after I assured him I wouldn't require vaccinations to be seen and that eighty percent of the treatments I did in my practice were completely holistic.

"Well, good morning Donald and Gracie," I said warmly as I held the door open for them. "Glad you decided to pay a visit!"

"Hello, Dr. Fox, thanks," Donald replied as he proceeded to tell me about his accident and the issues with his little companion.

"Oh my, it sounds like you've been through the wringer," I replied. "I can't believe you've been through all of that and yet you're up walking and even *working.*" Donald relayed how his pickup was smashed like an accordion between two semi-trailers and how it took several hours to extricate him from the wreckage. How he survived was totally an act of God.

Donald chuckled and assured me he and his wife were about as holistic as they could get, describing how they used a certain type of water system, homeopathics, home remedies, etc. for both themselves and all of their animals. He was convinced the only reason he was alive today was his strong belief in natural medicine.

"Well, I'm going to have you fill out some paperwork, Donald, and I'll get a weight on Gracie." As Donald sat down with clipboard and pen, I attempted to slip a leash on my patient. She uttered a low growl and "smiled" so that all of her big, beautiful canine teeth were visible. Her lips and jaws chattered with the warning, "Hey, back OFF!"

"Oh, wait, I'll help you," Donald interjected, "she doesn't like new people. Especially vets."

I had to laugh, because Gracie was the typical *don't-mess-with-me* type of terrier, and her menacing "smile" was pretty darn funny. Although I was certain she would bite me at the drop of a hat, I never let her intimidate me. In future visits, I would just laugh as her grumbling escalated to a high-pitched screech. Donald did a great job holding her when we had to trim her toenails and express her anal glands. Normally, I wouldn't let clients restrain their own dogs, but Gracie trusted her guardian and knew he was in charge.

I started the exam on Gracie by first assessing her neck mobility. I had her owner gently move her head and neck sideways, then up, then down. No problems there. Next, I had Donald hold her mouth shut while I palpated her spine, from tail to base of neck. She cringed a little when I got close to the neck. Since she was such an active little gal, I assumed she had perhaps injured something in her spine. Her temperature was slightly elevated, at 102.2 degrees. Next, I felt around on her chest and abdomen for any abnormalities in the mammary glands. A pea-sized nodule was felt in the far gland on the left side. I mentioned it to Donald and asked him if that was new. He hadn't been aware of any growths, so I told him he could monitor it for a few weeks, or the best suggestion was to have it surgically removed and biopsied. We discussed the fact that unspayed female dogs are more prone to mammary tumors, whether they're benign or malignant.

"Dr. Fox, I don't want to sound like a bad pet owner, but at her age, I don't want to put her through any surgery. I think it would be too hard on her."

"I can appreciate that, Donald, but here's the deal. She's not spayed. There is a good chance that Gracie can develop what we call a 'pyometra'. That means that the uterus gets infected which can quickly turn into a life-threatening situation. The other thing—and probably the more likely scenario—is that more growths can form in other nipples. If her condition is cancerous, the prognosis for long-term survival isn't good without surgery."

"I know, but she's had a good life so far. I hate the thought of taking her to a hospital and having her cut open. Plus, there's no guarantee that she won't have complications, right?"

"Of course Donald, I can't guarantee anything."

"Well, then, can we try something else besides regular medicine?" I could see the internal struggle within him. *Surgery. She's never been away from home—ever. What if she dies on the table? What if the cancer spreads because of the surgery? What if a pyometra never develops and this isn't cancer? Why put her through the misery and pain?*

"Donald, I don't want to put any pressure on you. I'm simply looking out for Gracie's well-being. I will support you in whatever decision you make. And yes, we can try to manage this issue with natural products and therapies."

"Good, because I'm not going to take her anywhere for surgery. I'm leaving it up to you to help her."

I secretly questioned his decision to let Gracie live out her life as she was. Perhaps the growth was actually benign and she would never develop an infected uterus. But as I got to know Donald better over the next few years, I commended his decision to take a totally natural route with Gracie.

We chose a course of essential oils (primarily boswellia sacra, copaiba, and lavender) for topical application on the nipple with the growth; a homeopathic tablet for liver support; whole-food supplements for immune and intestinal support. In addition, since Gracie had a slightly cloudy appearance to her eyes (which is more common in older dogs as the lens thickens), I started Gracie on one teaspoon of a commercially-prepared antioxidant juice with wolfberries, fruit juice extracts, and essential oils. To cover all bases, I prescribed an antibiotic for a few days since she was running a fever.

Four months later, Donald brought Gracie back to my office for a nail trim and anal gland expression. Today she seemed lethargic and stiff and was again running a low-grade fever. We pulled blood for a complete comprehensive blood panel and a Lyme disease test, but nothing out of ordinary showed up in the results. Her red and white cells counts were perfect. The only slight elevation was in one of her liver enzymes, but it wasn't elevated enough to make me concerned. The mass on Gracie's mammary gland had increased slightly in size and exuded a watery brown fluid when gently squeezed. I was concerned that the mass was cancerous since benign growths rarely have this kind of discharge. She also was leaking a bit of vaginal fluid and appeared to be coming into a heat cycle. I prepared several slides with discharge from both areas, stained them, and looked at them under the microscope. I saw some ugly-looking cells from the mammary gland; cells that appeared in clumps and were pretty suspicious of a carcinoma. I told Donald that I am indeed not a pathologist, but years of looking at slides like this made me pretty certain Gracie had cancer. Fortunately, the slide of her reproductive system fluid had cells you'd find in a normal heat cycle. There was no evidence of a pyometra, or cancer in the uterus.

"Donald, I'm going to again encourage you to get this mass taken off of Gracie. I don't like what I'm seeing under the microscope," I pleaded with my client. "We have a chance to get this under control since there is only one small mass. But left alone, I'm afraid it will spread."

"Dr. Fox, I said before, and I'll say it again, no surgery for my Gracie."

"Okay, you know I just have to give you my best advice and explain all options," I reiterated. "Let's tweak Gracie's protocol so we can get this whole thing slowed down."

Gracie gave me her best "smile" as I proceeded to apply frankincense, sandalwood, balsam fir, lavender, and blue spruce to her mammary gland. Donald admitted he'd only been putting the oils on about every other day, so we discussed the importance of getting them on twice daily *every single day.* Added to her protocol were two essential oil blends that would help balance out her female hormones.

Eight weeks later, I trimmed Gracie's toenails and expressed her anal glands. Amazingly, the mammary mass had shrunken greatly in size and there was no more brown fluid in the gland. Her heart and lungs sounded normal through the stethoscope. Even her eyes appeared bright and clear, with none of the cloudiness I'd seen several months earlier. I dispensed more of the homeopathic remedy for liver support and had Donald continue the same protocol of essential oils topically. He continued to give Gracie the antioxidant juice faithfully.

I didn't see Gracie until the following winter, in February of 2015. Donald and I had communicated via phone several times between appointments. He thought the tumor had gotten bigger, although Gracie was her normal, active, vivacious self. Today, I felt a "stalk" at the base of the tumor, which had grown to about two centimeters in diameter. Instead of having a smooth, round feel, it felt more like a small clump of cauliflower.

The brownish exudate had returned. We added citrus essential oils, such as grapefruit, orange, tangerine, and lemon due to their high levels of d-limonene, which is a potent anti-inflammatory. Donald continued to use the whole food powdered supplements mixed into Gracie's homemade diet of chicken, deer, and beef along with a variety of vegetables from their garden.

As usual, Gracie gave me her best smile and low grumble as I trimmed her nails and expressed her anal glands.

April 2015: no big changes in the tumor were noted. The products were holding the tumor back in size. We continued the same protocol.

June 2015: Gracie's tumor had changed in shape and size. This time, it appeared as a fluid-filled sac that hung down from her belly. Her heart and lungs sounded normal through the stethoscope. I instructed Donald to increase the frequency of the oils to four times daily.

August 2015: As I trimmed Gracie's nails and expressed her anal glands, she seemed more agitated than normal. Although the mass had shrunken somewhat and didn't hang down as much, I was concerned about metastasis to other organs. However, her lungs sounded clear as a bell and Gracie was still very active, running along Donald's tractor as he did his chores. At this time, I didn't add anything different. The tumor seemed to be halted in its growth.

January 2016: Donald brought Gracie in for her standard nail trim and anal gland expression. One of her rear toenails had become so long it had curled under and had embedded in the foot pad. I trimmed it out and applied lavender and cistus essential oils to help the wound heal. Donald mentioned that Gracie had slowed down greatly and preferred to sit on the tractor with him, rather than run beside it. Today when I examined Gracie, I found an enlarged lymph node in the back of her right rear leg, possibly indicative of cancer spreading throughout her body. However, she still had clear lungs and her weight had held steady throughout her journey with cancer.

July 2016: Gracie's tumor had exploded in growth over the past four weeks. I was shocked when I examined her —the tumor was a huge hanging sack of fluid and lumps—and it had started to ooze and drain from the skin on the underside. Blue and black spots covered the entire mass. It was one of the ugliest growths I'd ever seen. Another tumor was quickly growing in the gland just behind the original. Amazingly, Gracie was still active, eating well, and her old feisty self. I started Gracie on an oral antibiotic to reduce chances of infection from the lesions on the mass, and gave Donald "the talk."

"Gosh, this is so hard to bring up," I said hesitantly. "It's obvious we're losing this battle. You need to prepare for helping Gracie transition, whether you choose to have her put to sleep or let her go peacefully at home. If she is suffering relentlessly and we can't manage her comfort, it's time to let her go."

Donald voice quavered as he choked back tears. "I know. I get what you're saying, but…" I waited as he composed himself. "She still jumps up on the ATV and wants to go for rides. Even though she doesn't always want to eat, I find something that sparks her interest. I just can't let her go yet."

"I understand Donald, this is such a hard decision. I trust you'll know when it's time."

"Yes, Dr. Fox, I promise I won't let Gracie suffer."

A few weeks later, I talked with Donald on the phone. He told me the mass had ruptured, and Gracie was feeling good. The original tumor had dried up and was half the size it had grown to. But the second tumor had become very aggressive, growing quickly and turning "ugly" like the first. I told him to be aggressive with the oils and pray for Gracie's healing.

September 19, 2016: Donald called and said Gracie had quit eating for the past few days and that she was having labored breathing. He had scheduled an appointment to have Gracie euthanized the following morning. He felt she had completely given up, and was suffering. However, Gracie quietly and peacefully slipped into the afterlife later that evening, with Donald and his wife, Anna, petting and comforting her. Gracie was fifteen years of age.

* * * *

Author's note: Gracie's journey with cancer was a testimonial to her owner's intuition—that surgery and/or chemotherapy may have been detrimental to her—and his decision to support her with natural products gave her good quality of life until just a few weeks before her death. Donald allowed Gracie to pass naturally as long as he could manage her discomfort, which was minimal until the very end. It was an honor to have followed Gracie's progress for the three years after she developed cancer; the lessons learned from this journey are invaluable.

Chapter 19 – Helping Kota with Severe Arthritis

One of the most common medical issues that seems to dominate the requests for help from the alternative veterinary medicine world is arthritis. Though there are several forms of arthritis, it commonly boils down to inflammation that settles in the joints. After all, when you break down the word, "arthro" means joints, and "itis" simply means inflammation. Osteoarthritis, or DJD (degenerative joint disease) is the most common form of the oftentimes debilitating condition.

Kota, a kind, friendly chocolate Labrador mix, had suffered from significant joint issues all of her life. Her owners, Gary and Trudy, had adopted her from a shelter as a young puppy. She was the smallest of her litter—the runt; unfortunately, these puppies are commonly afflicted with various maladies. At a year of age, Kota had already exhibited signs of moderate to severe hip dysplasia, which progressed to the point where now, six years later, she had great difficulty even standing. Her guardians were worried sick. They loved her dearly and wanted to do everything they could for her, especially with natural products. The middle-aged couple had a passion for the Native American way of healing and sought the most holistic path they could for Kota.

I have to admit this dog had one of the worst cases of arthritis I'd ever seen. She had major atrophy (shrinking) of her rear leg muscles, making her legs appear abnormally skinny for her body. Every bone and joint was clearly visible through her moderately thick coat of fur. When she walked, her hind legs were so weak and/or painful that they crossed over each other frequently. The instability caused Kota to sway and wobble like she'd had a six-pack of beer injected into her bloodstream. It broke my heart to see such an advanced case of DJD because there would be little hope for even partial resolution of her condition.

"So has Kota ever had x-rays taken of her pelvis and hip joints?" I queried at our first appointment. I was asking as many detailed questions and writing as many notes as I could so a suitable protocol could be started.

"We had those done when she started limping several years ago. Haven't had any since," Gary responded. "They were pretty bad back then. The vet said the only hope for her was surgery. But we were going to have to take her to a specialty hospital for that. At the time, we didn't have the funds and the vet even said it might be too late because her hips were so bad."

I nodded in agreement as I sighed and leaned back in my chair. "I understand, Gary. It sounds like Kota had a rough enough start in life that even *with* surgery, it might not have made a difference. Here's the scoop. We know she has very advanced joint disease. We're not going to be able to "fix" that. What our goal will be is to give her as much quality of life as possible, and when we can't achieve that anymore, then we'll know we've done everything we can. Then it will be time to let her go."

"We know that, Dr. Fox," Trudy interjected, "and we appreciate your honesty. Our veterinarian back home is giving us a guilt trip for keeping her going. He said we should have put her to sleep two years ago. But she eats good, even tries to chase squirrels, and loves to lay on her foam bed and watch TV with us at night. I don't feel she's ready to be put down yet."

"You know your dog better than anyone else. You'll know when she's miserable and has given up. How do you get her up and down steps at home? I'm assuming she has at least a few to navigate to go out to potty?"

"Oh, Gary built a nice wooden ramp for her so she doesn't have to do any steps," Trudy replied. "We used to have to carry her, at least her back end, before he put in the ramp."

"Wonderful. Now let's talk about diet. What are you feeding her?"

"Well, we've been giving her Solid Gold, the Sundancer formula. We give her scrambled eggs as well."

"That's a pretty good food if we're comparing it to other dry kibble diets," I commented, "although we really need to get her on a partially cooked homemade diet or raw diet. If that isn't something you can do, then at least give her a portion of what you're cooking for dinner, such as lean cuts of roast or steak or unseasoned baked chicken. It's really important to get more nutrition into Kota."

The couple agreed to add more meat and fresh veggies into her diet. I suggested a commercially-prepared mineral supplement that they could add to her food daily. In my opinion, many joint diseases can be augmented with the addition of minerals. Magnesium deficiency can directly be associated with cartilage damage, and copper, zinc, manganese, and selenium tend to have anti-inflammatory effects in both human and animal scientific studies.

Kota's thyroid levels had always tested on the low-normal side, so I added a natural thyroid supplement in addition to a product containing all of the essential amino acids, MSM (naturally-occuring sulfur), vitamin E, B vitamins, CoQ10, and many other trace ingredients. Essential oils of oregano, thyme, basil, spruce, peppermint, copaiba, and wintergreen were mixed in combination and applied to Kota's spine and hips three times weekly. A homeopathic remedy for arthritis, and a whole food supplement for overall body support was chosen. Kota's owners at least had something to start with. This would be a difficult case and I was less than optimistic about any kind of real change.

A few months later, I rechecked Kota at her home, since the hour-long trip to my office was too much for the ailing canine. I liked the fact that I could see her in her own environment, which is a huge advantage with house calls. The ranch-style home was painted with warm brown hues and the entire yard exemplified Gary and Trudy's love for nature: an expansive garden, clumps of wildflowers throughout the yard, beautiful maple and oak trees lining the back of their one-acre lot. Native American decor adorned the split-rail fencing in front, and colorful ornaments hung on both sides of the garage doors. As I pulled in, Kota bounded through the back door and hurriedly ambled down the ramp to greet me.

"Wow, Kota, you are looking good girl!" I was shocked at how her mobility had improved since I'd last seen her. Not only was she moving more easily, but her fur had a shiny, smooth appearance I hadn't noticed before.

"Good morning Dr. Fox!" Trudy shouted. "Thanks for making

the trip over here! I see Kota is happy to meet you again."

I laughed and replied, "Well, not all my patients are always happy to see me. Glad she feels differently!

"Trudy, whatever you and Gary are doing for this girl, keep it up. She is so much stronger than she was two months ago. I have to admit, I'm really impressed with her progress." I didn't want to tell the couple that I held out little hope for Kota. No sense in dwelling on what *might not* have happened.

"We're taking walks around the block several times a day, Dr. Fox," Trudy related with a smile. "Even the neighbors are amazed at how well she is doing!"

Kota's back legs were still spindly for her body size, but there was a small amount of muscle that had started to build over the bony protuberances I'd seen earlier. Even though she was still weak, the progress she was making was truly remarkable.

Over the course of the next few years, Kota continued to rally. Trudy and Gary were faithful with treating her with essential oils, good diet, exercise, supplements, and the homeopathic remedy. Kota was now being walked at least a mile twice daily, with little discomfort.

* * * *

At this writing, Kota is now eleven years young and still going strong. The power of faith and natural healing is utterly amazing. Kota is living proof of a true miracle.

Chapter 20 – Stormy's Emotional Release

Losing one of our animals has always been one of the toughest times for me. I have gotten better with it over the years, knowing in my heart I'll see my beautiful babies in heaven one day... it's still darn tough to let go and say goodbye. As you might wonder, do animals go through a similar grieving process?

The tears flowed for months, probably even a few years, after I lost my two lovely Arabian horses, Ty and Ibn. Their bond was so incredibly close that they died twenty-four hours apart from each other. Ibn, a brilliant white gelding who was full of life and loved to play tricks on his human friends, developed unresolvable complications from Cushing's disease. Through various medications, diligent attention to his feet from a good friend and certified journeyman farrier, Raymond Legel, and surgery at Iowa State University, we were able to manage his pain and give him fairly good quality of life until he turned twenty-one years of age. This was prior to my introduction to holistic medicine, and I'm convinced I could have helped Ibn greatly with the use of herbs, essential oils, and changes in his nutrition.

Ty and Ibn had been buddies for almost a decade, sharing favorite grazing spots, traveling to horse shows together, engaging in mutual back scratching, and just enjoying each other's company. When one horse happened to move out of sight of the other, frantic galloping and whinnying ensued until the other returned. Stormy, the third gelding we acquired, became part of the family, and the three horses quickly developed a lasting companionship.

Ty, my tall chestnut Arabian who I "retired" from the show ring and rode in dressage clinics afterward, had just turned twenty-five years old. On the dreaded day when Ibn gave up on life, Ty became fatally sick and joined his buddy on the other side just twenty-four hours later.

It is my solid belief that Ty did not want to live without his best friend, as he had never been sick a day in his long and happy life. (I write about this in detail in my first book, *The Infinite Bond*).

Poor Stormy—he did not handle the loss of his two best friends well. We immediately "borrowed" a friend's horse to keep Stormy company; all was well for a while, until he started to age prematurely and also develop signs of Cushing's disease. Not only did he show the physical signs, but he acted depressed and detached from his pasture mate, Pal. As Stormy's weight plummeted and he turned into a "little old man" in front of me, I became very worried. I mentioned this to a large animal colleague of mine, Dr. Merle, and he suggested that I have an "emotional release session" done on him. I'd never heard of such a thing, as this happened before I was into alternative medicine. Briefly, Dr. Merle explained that the procedure involves letting an animal (or person) inhale or have specific essential oils applied topically in a peaceful, serene atmosphere. Essential oils have the ability to calm and relax the mind, allowing the non-beneficial emotions to be released. A lot of the success of this therapy lies in how easily the patient can "let go." That's why animals seem to be so easy to work with in comparison with humans—they have no preconceived ideas and no hangups to speak of—and the results are oftentimes amazing. I desperately wanted to do anything I could to help Stormy, whom I affectionately nicknamed "Beautiful Boy."

Dr. Merle helped line up several "healers," who used principles of Reiki and other energy modalities for the session. After briefing the team of energy workers headed by William, the group gathered around Stormy and gently stroked and rubbed his neck until they felt him relax. William chose an essential oil blend that was touted to instill courage and confidence. He applied a few drops to Stormy's neck, then allowed him to smell it directly from the bottle. The gentle gelding inhaled deeply. Next, William took another bottle from his case, removed the cap, and let Stormy sniff. This time, he yawned widely, which I learned was a sign of releasing. For the next half an hour, various oils were given, either aromatically or topically, depending on Stormy's preference. If he turned away from an oil, the oil was not used.

At one point deep into the session, he dropped his nose closely to the ground. Stormy blinked rapidly and he began making chewing motions with his mouth. His facial muscles writhed into strange contortions. One of the healers said quietly, "Oh, poor boy, he's bawling his eyes out." I was amazed; it truly looked like he was sobbing. For five full minutes Stormy continued this behavior while the group of healers continued to place oils that were calming and soothing on his back. The healers continued to lay their hands on Stormy as more oils were applied over the next thirty minutes.

I was loosely holding the lead rope. I whispered to Dr. Merle, "When will you know he's done releasing?"

William overhead the question and answered, "He'll let us know. Just watch."

A few minutes after orange oil was dropped onto his back, Stormy suddenly backed up with lightning speed, ripping the lead rope out of my hands. He spun and took off galloping across the pasture. The bay gelding stopped, dropped, and rolled several times in the soft dirt. Stormy leaped up, shook himself off furiously, then exploded into a full-blown run. After the second pass across the pasture, he halted. *This* time, he looked just like the young and vibrant Stormy I remembered so well. He stood like a statue, with his head and neck held majestically high in the air and his tail curled up over his back. He blew through his nostrils, making a shrill whistle, then bucked in place and again took off galloping.

Tears of relief filled my eyes as I witnessed the incredible metamorphosis in my beautiful boy. The old Stormy was back! His eyes were full of life and expression again. How I wished I had known about this therapy earlier, when Stormy needed it most!

Dr. Merle made me aware that some animals, as well as people, can continue to release these feelings for days or even weeks after the initial therapy. Sometimes a second session needs to be conducted, especially if there was a lot of trauma in one's life.

My beautiful boy continued to thrive for the next several years. Then, at twenty-one years of age, he again began to exhibit symptoms of Cushing's disease: minor flare-ups of the laminitis he experienced prior to his first emotional release; excess fat deposits on his rump, neck, and shoulders; shedding out late in the summer, only to grow thick hair just a few weeks later. Essential oils, a whole food metabolic supplement, and careful attention to Stormy's diet managed his condition well, until the next summer.

At that time, Stormy had little tolerance for the heat and humidity. We placed large utility fans in the corncrib and in the lower part of the dairy barn to keep him and his buddy, Pal, cool. Stormy sprouted white hairs on his muzzle, making him look older than what he actually was. In June, I had to leave home for several days as I was invited to speak at an international essential oils conference in Salt Lake City. Severe weather had been predicted for a good portion of the week, and as always, I was concerned for the horses' safety. There is really no safe place for humans and animals to be when bad weather hits; we just leave it up to our horses to "know" where it's best for them to be, inside a shelter or outside. One of my friends lost four of her five horses in a horrible EF-5 tornado—the most violent tornado rating there is. The surviving horse ran out of his shelter and sandwiched himself against the cement wall in the back of the shelter, seeming to sense that was the safest place to be.

To my utter shock and grief, our Beautiful Boy passed away quietly and peacefully of a major heart attack or aneurysm two days after I left home. My husband said he was perfectly fine at 9:00 p.m. the night before; Gary had been petting him as he drank from the water tank. There had been no storms; the weather had been unusually quiet. The next morning, our precious Stormy lay at the bottom of the pasture, facing the timber where Ty and Ibn were buried...

It is my heartfelt thought that Stormy felt a huge void after the deaths of his best buddies. Though the emotional release sessions helped him, the loss was still there. I believe Stormy "waited" until I left to let himself pass peacefully into the next realm. There is much more to the story, which I've written about in my first book, *The Infinite Bond*. The book describes the tremendous connection the horses had, and how they helped me through a dark time in my own life.

As a result of witnessing my beloved horses' deaths and their emotional ties, I speak about this perception at various conferences and seminars. If you need convincing that animals do have emotions, I encourage you to explore this more.

Barb Fox DVM

AUTHOR | SPEAKER | CONSULTANT

www.barbfoxdvm.com

Acknowledgements

To all of the wonderful, loving pet parents I've met with, thank you for all you do for your beautiful animal friends and for keeping an open mind.

To William Lansing and Dr. Merle Kuennen, thank you for teaching me about the wonderful world of essential oils and how to use them for emotional releasing.

To Laura Ashton, thank you for your editing skills and talent in putting this book together.

To Ray Legel, certified journeyman farrier, for your incredible knowledge, persistence, and diligence in working with Ibn's foot issues, thank you from the bottom of my heart.

To my husband, Gary, who strongly encouraged me to write this book, thank you, and I love you more than you'll ever know.

To the practitioners who believed in my strength and my health, and who helped pull me through some very difficult health challenges, I love you!! Thank you for your unwavering support and care.

Most of all, I am very grateful for the beautiful animals I've been blessed to help. The animals provided me with some of the best education in the universe. Their unconditional love, beliefs, and lessons are immeasurable.

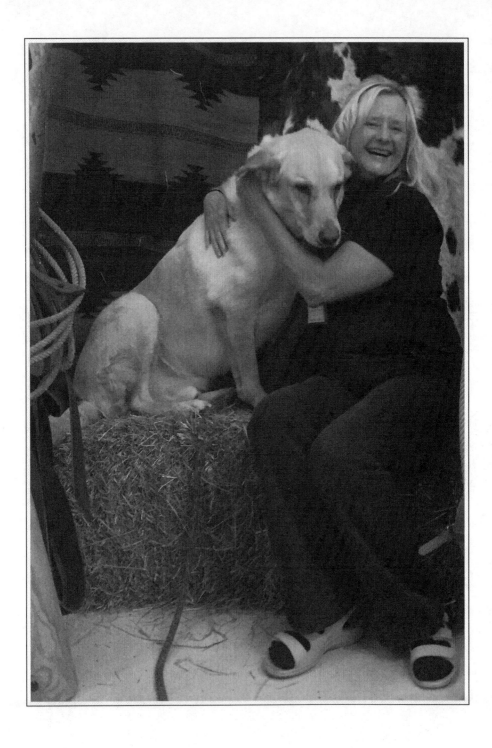

About the Author

Dr. Barb Fox graduated from Iowa State University's College of Veterinary Medicine in 1994. She worked in various practices in northeast Iowa and eventually opened her own mobile veterinary clinic. In 2007, after being diagnosed with a potentially fatal medical condition, she turned to alternative and complementary medicine instead of choosing a strictly conventional treatment plan. Thrilled with the results, she passionately began a course of education and research into holistic modalities for her own animal patients.

After years of incorporating pure, unadulterated essential oils, nutritional supplements, homeopathic remedies, massage therapy, and quantum physics principles with her patients, she has become a strong advocate for a holistic approach to health and wellness. Dr. Fox is a firm believer in the mind-body-spirit connection, so much of her work involves addressing underlying emotional issues that can impede physical healing.

Dr. Fox has spoken on various holistic health topics pertaining to people and animals at national and regional conferences, and teaches many local classes on safe and effective usage of essential oils. She is a member of the American Holistic Veterinary Medical Association and the Veterinary Medical Aromatherapy Association.

In her spare time, Dr. Fox enjoys rock hunting, hiking, and spending time in the mountains of Colorado. She and her husband Gary live in beautiful northeast Iowa with their two horses, Chaser and Pal, and their eight house kitties.

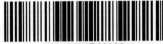

Made in the USA
San Bernardino, CA
14 January 2019